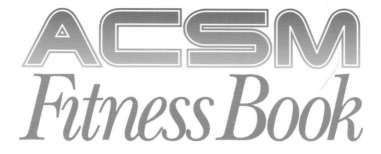

ACSM
Fitness Book

American College of Sports Medicine

Leisure Press
Champaign, Illinois

Library of Congress Cataloging-in Publication Data

ACSM fitness book / American College of Sports Medicine.
    p. cm.
    Includes index.
    ISBN 0-88011-460-6
    1. Exercise. 2. Physical fitness--Testing. I. American College
of Sports Medicine. II. Title: Fitness book.
GV481.A32 1992
613.7'1--dc20   91- 40288
                                         CIP

ISBN: 0-88011-460-6

Copyright © 1992 by American College of Sports Medicine

Developmental Editor: Holly Gilly
Assistant Editors: Elizabeth Bridgett,
   Dawn Levy, and Kari Nelson
Copyeditor: Molly Bentsen
Proofreader: Kari Nelson
Production Director: Ernie Noa
Typesetter: Kathy Boudreau-Fuoss
Text Design: Keith Blomberg
Text Layout: Denise Lowry

Cover Photo: Wilmer Zehr
Cover Design: Jack Davis
Cartoons: Dick Flood
Anatomical Drawings: Roger Phillips
Factoids: Doug Burnett
Interior Photos: Photo Concepts/John
   Kilroy
Producer: Mandarin Offset

Leisure Press books are available at special discounts for bulk purchase for sales promotions, premiums, fund-raising, or educational use. Special editions or book excerpts can also be created to specification. For details, contact the Special Sales Manager at Leisure Press.

Printed in Hong Kong

10 9 8 7 6 5 4 3

Leisure Press
A Division of Human Kinetics Publishers
Box 5076, Champaign, IL 61825-5076
1-800-747-4457

Canada: Human Kinetics Publishers, P.O. Box 2503, Windsor, ON N8Y 4S2
1-800-465-7301 (in Canada only)

Europe: Human Kinetics Publishers (Europe) Ltd., P.O. Box IW14, Leeds LS16 6TR
England
0532-781708

Australia: Human Kinetics Publishers, P.O. Box 80, Kingswood 5062,
South Australia
618-374-0433

New Zealand: Human Kinetics Publishers New Zealand, P.O. Box 105-231,
Auckland 1
(09) 309-2259

Contents

Foreword

The evidence continues to mount: Regular physical activity is an effective preventive health measure. Physical fitness, resulting from an active rather than a sedentary lifestyle, has value in and of itself. People who exercise regularly report an improved sense of overall well-being. But from a health perspective, physical activity—together with a balanced and prudent diet—appears to be one of the most important positive steps that we can take to reduce the likelihood of developing coronary heart disease, reduce the risk of some forms of cancer, and prevent and manage adult-onset diabetes. Likewise, it is associated with lowered levels of blood pressure, obesity, chronic back pain, cigarette smoking, lost work time from disability, and overall health-care costs.

For all these reasons, the *ACSM Fitness Book* readers can understand my concern to get Americans up and moving. A principal priority for improving the health of the American people during the coming decade, as spelled out in Healthy People 2000, our health promotion agenda for the nation, is physical activity and fitness. I commend the American College of Sports Medicine for sponsoring the development of this exercise guide. I urge its readers to become users and to enjoy the benefits of physical fitness and improved health.

Louis W. Sullivan, MD
Secretary of Health and Human Services

Preface

With all the books on exercise and fitness, many by famous entertainers, on bookstore shelves, why is this one different?

The *ACSM Fitness Book* is the product of the American College of Sports Medicine (ACSM), a group of exercise science professionals and scholars dedicated to furthering their knowledge about exercise and passing that knowledge on to the public. ACSM counts among its more than 13,000 members the world's top scientists, physicians, educators, and fitness professionals.

A team of these experts created the *ACSM Fitness Book* and its scientifically sound, effective method for beginning an exercise program. It is not a book for the already-fit. Rather, it is for people who, whatever their motivation, are ready to begin exercising, but need a game plan to get started.

True fitness includes four components—cardiorespiratory fitness, muscular strength and endurance, flexibility, and healthy body composition—and the ACSM Fitness Program helps you improve all four. Our emphasis is on exercise that is *healthy* and *individualized*. Using a simple four-part assessment, the ACSM Fitness Test, you determine your current level of fitness. Then following step-by-step instructions, you create an exercise program suited exactly for you, updating it as your fitness improves.

We applaud you for considering the decision to begin exercising. It will take commitment, but the results are worth the effort. We at ACSM would like to do our part to help you reach your goals. Good luck!

W. Larry Kenney, PhD, FACSM
Associate Professor, Pennsylvania State University
Editor

About the ACSM Fitness Book *Writing Team*

Editor

W. Larry Kenney, PhD, FACSM, is Associate Professor of Applied Physiology at Penn State University. He is certified as an ACSM Exercise Specialist™ and as an ACSM Program Director™ who was awarded the prestigious ACSM New Investigator Award in 1987 for his research in environmental physiology.

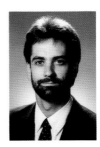

Writers

Susan M. Puhl, PhD, is Assistant Professor of Exercise and Sport Science at Penn State University and is certified as an ACSM Health/Fitness Instructor™. Her expertise is in exercise gerontology with a specific research interest in methods of analyzing body composition.

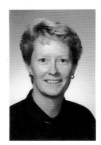

Patricia M. Kenney, MS, is certified as an ACSM Exercise Specialist™. She is Fitness Coordinator and an instructor in the Department of Exercise and Sport Science at Penn State University. Her area of specialization is developing and administrating fitness programs for adults.

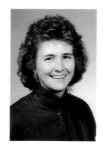

Arch F. Moore, EdD, is Professor of Health and Physical Education at Indiana University of Pennsylvania. His area of specialty is exercise prescription, including rehabilitative exercise for cardiac patients.

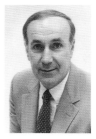

IIII *Chapter 1*

Why Begin an Exercise Program?

The best reason for beginning an exercise program is a genuine desire to improve your health and fitness. By reading this book, you're taking an important first step. The decision to take charge of your exercise lifestyle is a vital one, and an appropriate program can help you do it correctly. Exercise science experts from the American College of Sports Medicine (ACSM) have created this book to help you develop your own healthy exercise program.

The ACSM Fitness Program is designed for the beginning exerciser. The activities, developed by exercise science professionals, are meant for adults who may have been inactive for a few or many years. Even if you consider yourself to be very unfit or you haven't exercised since you left school, the ACSM Fitness Program can help you improve your health and physical fitness. Best of all, the program takes you *gradually* through a progressive set of exercises. You'll find that exercise need not hurt to be good for you!

If you have already made a commitment to improve your health through exercise and are exercising regularly, our fitness assessments will help you determine whether the ACSM Fitness Program is right for you. If the assessments indicate that you're ready for a more vigorous exercise program, chapter 6, "The Next Step," will help you select an appropriate and safe one.

Why Should You Exercise?

Exercise is something that you do for yourself. Regardless of who may have suggested that you begin exercising, the choice to do it is a personal one.

Why do you want to exercise? A list follows to help you identify your reasons. Rate the degree to which each statement applies to you by writing *high*, *moderate*, or *low* in the blank next to the item. Write any additional reasons in the space at the end of the list.

Why I Want to Exercise

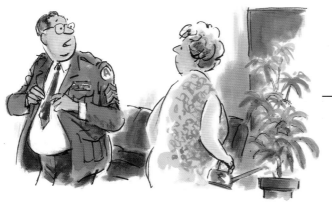

_____ I feel out of shape and want to improve my fitness.

_____ I've put on some extra weight.

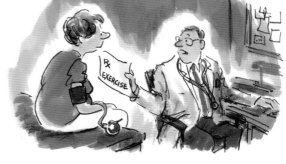

_____ My doctor suggested that I start exercising.

_____ I want to expand my social activities.

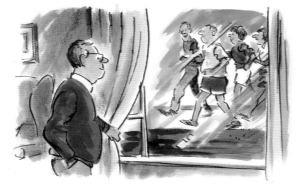

_____ I want to feel better and have more energy.

Additional reasons:

_____   _____

_____   _____

_____   _____

There are many reasons to exercise. Whatever yours are, you can look forward to several important benefits from a regular fitness program.

What You Can Expect From Regular Exercise

By being a regular participant in an exercise program, you'll improve not only your physical health, but your mental health as well. The lists that follow show how regular exercise contributes to a healthier heart and an improved outlook on life.

A Healthier Heart

- An increase in the amount of blood your heart can pump

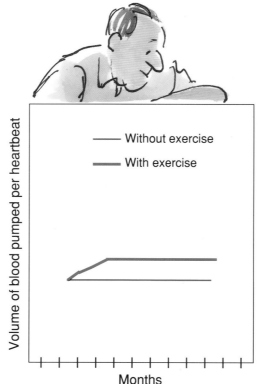

- A lower heart rate when your body is at rest

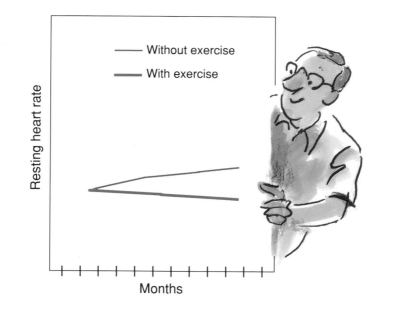

- Improved levels of cholesterol in your blood

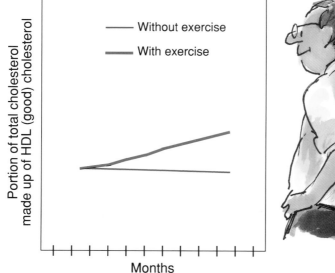

- Lower blood pressure

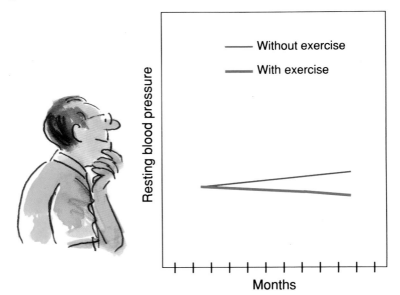

- Reduced body fat

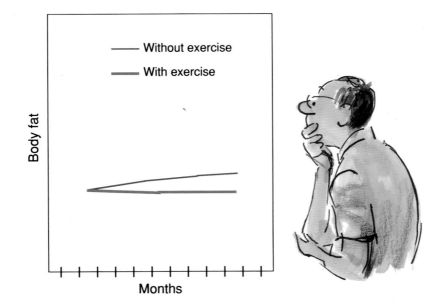

An Improved Outlook on Life

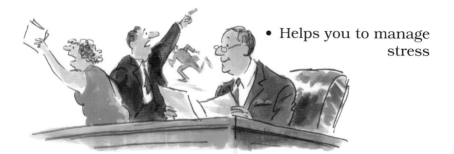

• Helps you to manage stress

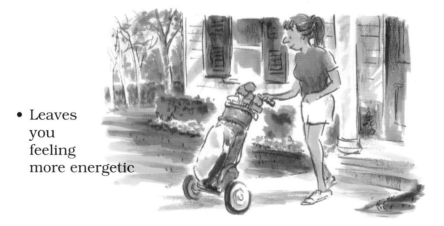

• Leaves you feeling more energetic

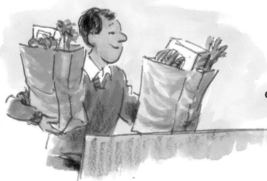

• Lets you more easily complete daily chores

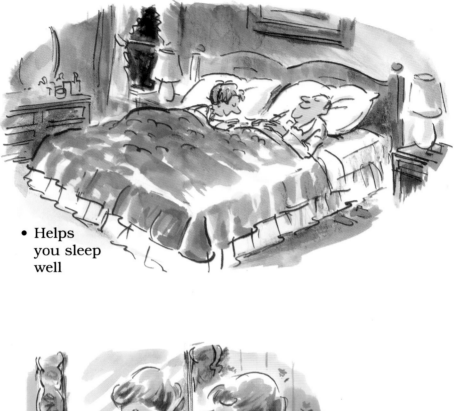

• Helps
you sleep
well

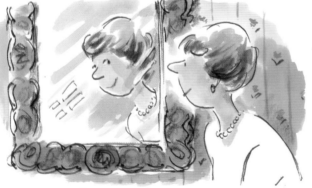

• Improves
your
self-image

As you can see, regular exercise can have far-reaching effects. At this point, you may be wondering, "Just what do I have to do to get all these benefits?" To answer that question, let's look at what fitness really means.

What Is Fitness?

Physical fitness refers to your ability to carry out daily tasks without being overly tired. People who are fit have energy not only to complete everyday work, but also to participate in planned and unplanned activities outside the home or other workplace.

Physical fitness actually has four components:

- Cardiorespiratory fitness—the heart's ability to pump blood and deliver oxygen throughout your body
- Muscular fitness—the strength and endurance of your muscles
- Flexibility—the ability to move your joints freely and without pain through a wide range of motion
- Body composition—concerned with the portion of your body weight made up of fat

Because fitness has different components, no one exercise alone will let you achieve total fitness. The *ACSM Fitness Book* provides you with an exercise *program*, combining different types of exercises to improve your fitness in all four areas.

Cardiorespiratory Fitness

The ACSM Fitness Program uses walking to improve cardiorespiratory fitness. Walking is an excellent exercise because it involves most of the large muscles of the body, puts minimal stress on joints, does not require expensive equipment, and can be done almost anywhere.

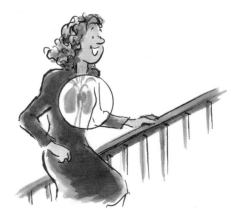

Muscular Strength and Endurance

Muscular fitness includes both strength (how much weight you can safely lift) and endurance (how many times you can lift or how long you can hold an object without fatigue). It is essential to many activities of your daily life, whether lifting a toddler or pushing a lawnmower. The ACSM Fitness Program uses a variety of exercises to improve both the strength and endurance of the major muscles of your upper and lower body.

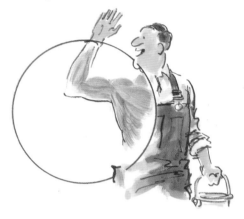

Flexibility

Flexibility is important for you to perform tasks that require reaching, twisting and turning your body, and moving objects. Hip flexibility, for example, is important to preventing lower back pain. A number of stretching exercises will help improve the flexibility of your body's major joints.

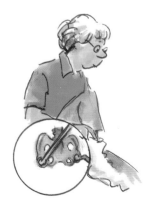

Body Composition

Your level of body fat can affect your risk of developing health problems. Too much fat puts extra weight strain on your joints and increases your risk of getting many diseases, including heart disease, high blood pressure, and diabetes. Too little body fat is also associated with your body's not functioning at its best. Body weight alone, though, is not a reliable indicator of body composition. A tall, heavy person may actually have a lot of muscle and be relatively healthy. And, a short, thin person may in fact have a high percentage of body fat, thus increasing health risks. In the ACSM Fitness Program, regular walking is the means to controlling body composition.

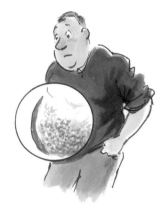

It's Easy to Get Fit!

The ACSM Fitness Program is designed to improve your overall fitness without being painful or overly stressful. The program emphasizes moderate exercise and gradual progressions. Exercise of moderate intensity done on a regular basis is more beneficial to your health than vigorous exercise done only occasionally. And, contrary to what you might have thought, exercise doesn't have to hurt to help.

Getting Ready for Exercise

T he activities in the *ACSM Fitness Book* are designed for adults of all ages who want to begin exercising. For most people, physical activity should not pose any problem or hazard, and no medical clearance is necessary.

Before You Begin

Before you begin your exercise program, however, take a few minutes to answer the questions in the Preparticipation Checklist on the next page. If you answer "yes" to any, we advise you to seek medical advice about the type of activity that is safe and appropriate for you *before* going any further with this program.

It will also be helpful for you to set some goals as you begin a fitness program. Good goals can help motivate you to stick with your exercise program and challenge you to push yourself that little bit harder. And it's a great feeling to set a goal and watch yourself achieve it! Refer back to the reasons you identified on pages 2 and 3 for beginning an exercise program,

Preparticipation Checklist

	Yes	No
1. Has a doctor ever said you have heart trouble?	——	——
2. Do you suffer frequently from chest pains?	——	——
3. Do you often feel faint or have spells of severe dizziness?	——	——
4. Has a doctor ever said your blood pressure was too high?	——	——
5. Has a doctor ever told you that you have a bone or joint problem, such as arthritis, that has been or could be aggravated by exercise?	——	——
6. Are you over age 65 and not accustomed to any exercise?	——	——
7. Are you taking any prescription medications, such as those for heart problems or high blood pressure?	——	——
8. Is there a good physical reason not mentioned here that you should not follow an activity program?	——	——

If you answer "yes" to any question, we advise you to consult with your physician before beginning an exercise program.

Note: From the PAR-Q Validation Report (modified version) by the British Columbia Department of Health, D.M. Chisholm, M.I. Collins, W. Davenport, N. Gruber, L.L. Kulak, 1975, *British Columbia Medical Journal*, 17.

then set goals that relate to those reasons. As you set your goals, follow these guidelines:

- Make your goals challenging, but realistic. For example, if it presently takes you 13 minutes to walk a mile it would be a more appropriate beginning goal to walk a mile in 11 minutes rather than in 8 minutes.

- Set specific, not general, goals. Don't set a goal "to improve muscular strength." Instead aim, for example, to increase the number of push-ups you can do at once from 10 to 15.
- Set goals that you can reach within a time period that is short enough to keep you motivated. Rather than setting a goal of losing 35 pounds this year, set one to lose 3 pounds this month.

Take a few minutes to think about your personal goals. After you've identified some, write them down here. Then as you continue in your exercise program, your list will help remind you how much you have achieved.

Personal Exercise Goals	
Date	Goal
———	—————————————————————
———	—————————————————————
———	—————————————————————
———	—————————————————————
———	—————————————————————
———	—————————————————————
———	—————————————————————
———	—————————————————————

Three Simple Steps to Fitness

The ACSM Fitness Program is designed to help you take the guesswork out of planning a safe, effective exercise routine with its simple 3-step approach to developing and maintaining fitness:

1. Find out where you are.
2. Build a program to get to where you want to be.
3. Check your progress.

Step 1. Find Out Where You Are

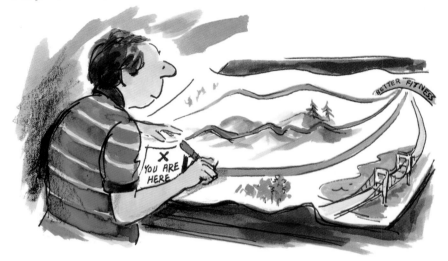

In order to exercise effectively and efficiently, it is important to know your current fitness status. Otherwise, you might choose an exercise program that is too difficult or too easy for you. In chapter 3, you'll take a simple 4-part test—the ACSM Fitness Test—to help you determine where you are in each fitness area. The assessments test the four components of physical fitness described in chapter 1.

Three parts of the ACSM Fitness Test can be completed in your own home. The walking part of the test can be done on any flat, measured walking surface, such as

- a neighborhood school or college track,
- a YMCA or YWCA,
- a community fitness center, or
- a sidewalk along a flat street (you'd need to measure this one yourself).

Ask someone to help you with the test or, better yet, to take the test with you so you can help each other.

To take the ACSM Fitness Test, it's best that you wear comfortable clothes and snug but comfortable shoes. Sweat clothes, shorts, T-shirts, and exercise tights are all appropriate clothing, but any loose, elastic-waist slacks and loose-fitting (especially across the shoulders) shirt or blouse will do. Sneakers or walking shoes are best for the walking part of the test, but any flat comfortable shoes are fine.

To perform the ACSM Fitness Test, you'll need to gather or borrow these items:

- A watch with a second hand (or a stopwatch)
- A ruler
- A body weight scale
- A yardstick
- Adhesive tape (any type)

Once you've gathered the items and are ready for the test, you (and a friend if possible) will do a few warm-up exercises before you begin (we provide appropriate exercises before each part of the test). The warm-up is important to any exercise session. It allows your heart rate and breathing to increase gradually, loosens your muscles, and warms your body so that you can exercise more safely. Your test results will also be better if you are properly warmed up. After you've done the warm-up exercises, you'll be ready to take

Warming-Up Safely & Effectively

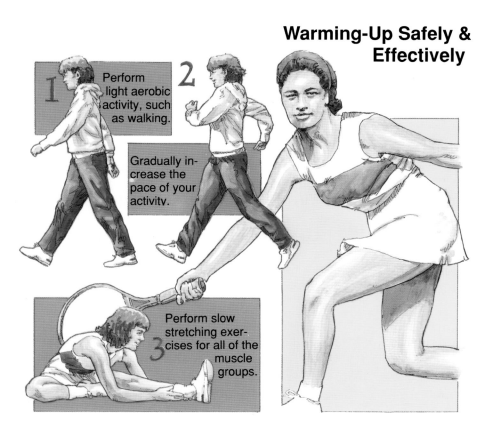

1 Perform light aerobic activity, such as walking.

Gradually increase the pace of your activity.

2

Perform slow stretching exercises for all of the muscle groups.

3

the ACSM Fitness Test described in chapter 3. When you've completed the test, you'll assign yourself points based on the results from each component.

Step 2. Build a Program to Get to Where You Want to Be

Your personal ACSM Fitness Program is based on your scores in each of the four fitness components. You'll use the scores to build an individual, color-coded exercise program. You may find, for example, that your test results indicate you're at a higher level of fitness in the cardiorespiratory component than the flexibility component. That's okay! When you assemble your program you'll choose the exercises that correspond to your fitness level for each component. That way, you can be sure that the exercises in the program are neither too hard nor too easy for your health and safety.

Once you've completed the ACSM Fitness Test and determined the colors to which you belong (for each fitness component), you'll be ready to build your exercise program. Chapter 5 provides easy-to-follow, day-by-day exercise schedules for each of the four colors, or levels.

Each level of the program takes you through 6 weeks of activity and includes exercises to improve all of the components of physical fitness. Each daily schedule includes specific exercises for you to complete.

To begin, you'll assemble a personalized version of the ACSM Fitness Program based on your scores from the ACSM Fitness

Test. You'll start at the appropriate level for each fitness component and continue until you successfully complete the entire program. When you finish one level of the program, you'll be instructed how to proceed to the next. You'll continue moving up until you've completed all levels of the program or until you've reached your fitness goals. Your fitness will be steadily improving! And it will be happening in a safe, enjoyable manner.

Step 3.   Check Your Progress

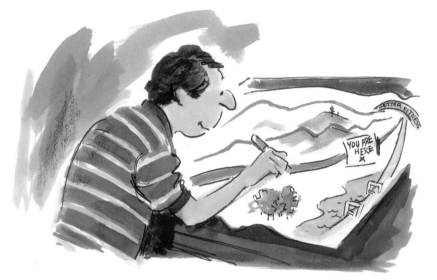

Keeping track of your progress in your ACSM Fitness Program is like checking the highway signs on a cross-country trip—it helps you know exactly where you are.

Along with the exercise programs in chapter 5, you'll find record sheets for tracking your exercise progress. Keeping records takes only a few seconds, but it's very important to your total fitness program. It takes the guesswork out of trying to remember what you did and how you felt each time you exercised. Each time you record your progress, you show yourself how far you've come. You'll also want to refer back periodically to the goals you've set (see page 15) to determine when you reach them. If you have met a goal, set a new one. It is easier to stay with your exercise program when you can see the progress you've made.

We hope you can see how easy it will be for you to use this book and to participate in the ACSM Fitness Program. We've done the planning for you, so that you can put all of your energy into improving your fitness.

Assessing Your Fitness: The ACSM Fitness Test

After reading this far, you should be familiar with the components of physical fitness. Now it's time to discover more about *your* fitness level.

This chapter describes the ACSM Fitness Test*, a compilation of four assessments to evaluate your current fitness level. The test is not time-consuming and is very easy to perform. You should enjoy the challenge, and the results will tell you much about your physical fitness.

The Importance of Assessing Your Fitness Level

Once you begin to exercise, you will be eager to learn about your improvement. You will begin to feel better, but there's much more to it. Numerous scientific studies indicate that regular exercise produces a variety of important physical changes. These changes are often hard to recognize because

---

*The ACSM Fitness Test is a compilation of four measures to help you evaluate your current fitness level. The individual tests were developed by other organizations whom we acknowledge at each test. The compilation is *not to be considered an official fitness test developed by ACSM.*

they occur gradually. For this reason, consider taking the ACSM Fitness Test regularly, every few months. This will help you not only to identify your rate of progress, but also to understand the level of effort required to make positive physical conditioning changes. As your score improves you will enjoy a great feeling of accomplishment and satisfaction.

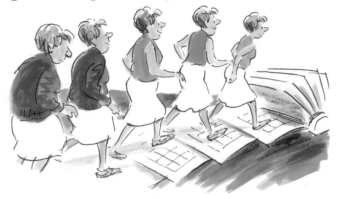

Is the ACSM Fitness Test the Same for Everyone?

The test is the same for every adult, regardless of gender, age, or activity level. However, the results will differ according to those categories. Standards have been developed to account for this, so that, for example, a 60-year-old is not compared with a 40-year-old, nor a man with a woman.

Your results reflect accepted standards for persons of your own age and gender. But the most important person with whom you should compare your results is *you*. This will allow you to see clear improvements in fitness as your program progresses.

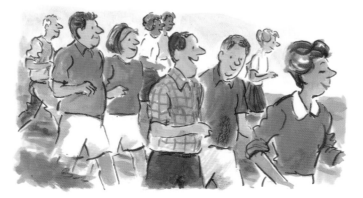

The Significance of Each Test Component

You have learned about the four fitness components. A high-fit person will score more points for the four components than a low-fit person, but many people will have varying scores. A good score in one category does not balance out a poor score in another. Your ultimate goal is to score well on all of the assessments.

Four Components of Fitness

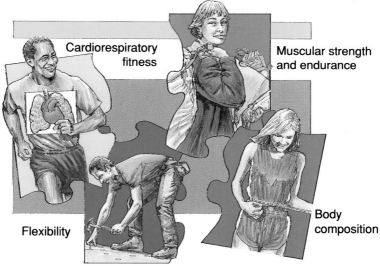

Cardiorespiratory fitness

Muscular strength and endurance

Flexibility

Body composition

ACSM Fitness Test Components

Described here are the four components of the ACSM Fitness Test. Each part has step-by-step instructions that are easy to follow and will help you perform the assessment properly. If you have recruited a friend to assist you, she or he can help with your body positioning and confirm that you are doing each part of the test correctly.

Fitness Component	*Assessment*
Cardiorespiratory fitness	Rockport one-mile walking test
Muscular strength and endurance	Push-up test
Flexibility	Modified sit-and-reach test
Body composition	Body mass index

Now you are ready to begin the ACSM Fitness Test.

Part I: Cardiorespiratory Fitness
Rockport One-Mile Walking Test

Equipment:

A watch with a second hand or a stopwatch

Preparation

1. Practice taking your pulse to determine your heart rate. This is not difficult, but it re- quires some practice. Your heart rate will be recorded in beats per minute. Using your index and middle fingers, locate your pulse at the base of your wrist or at the side of your neck near the Adam's apple (see Figure 3.1).

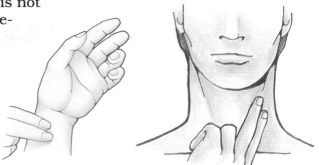

Figure 3.1   Heart rate (pulse) sites.

Determining Your Heart Rate

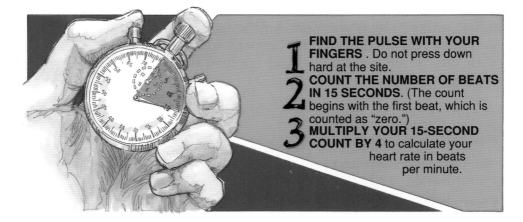

1 FIND THE PULSE WITH YOUR FINGERS . Do not press down hard at the site.

2 COUNT THE NUMBER OF BEATS IN 15 SECONDS. (The count begins with the first beat, which is counted as "zero.")

3 MULTIPLY YOUR 15-SECOND COUNT BY 4 to calculate your heart rate in beats per minute.

2. Do not eat, smoke, or drink coffee or tea for at least 2 hours before the test. In addition, don't participate in vigorous activity on the previous day.

3. Wear loose-fitting clothing that allows you to exercise comfortably. Your shoes should be suited to walking.

4. Find a place where you can walk for one mile on a level surface (see page 16 for some suggestions).

Procedure

1. Warm up thoroughly. You may start by walking slowly and gradually increasing your pace until you feel warm or begin to perspire. Recommended warm-up exercises are also shown.

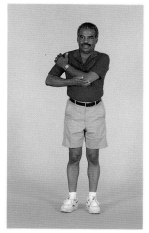
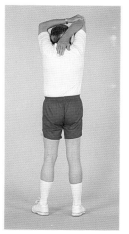
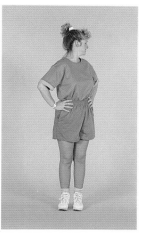

Shoulder Stretch   Triceps Stretch   Upper Body Twists

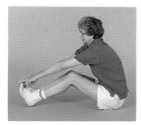
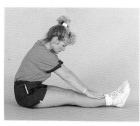

Calf and Hamstring   Seated Toe Touch
Stretch

2. Note the time or start the stopwatch and begin walking.

3. Stop walking after one mile, check your watch, and record your time to the nearest minute. _____ min. Add one minute to your time for every 25 pounds you weigh

over 125 pounds (for women) or 170 pounds (men). Subtract one minute from your time for every 25 pounds you weigh under 125 (women) or 170 (men). Record your adjusted time here. _____ min.

4. Immediately locate your pulse, take a 15-second count, and multiply by 4.

5. Record your heart rate in beats per minute. _____ bpm

Results

1. Select the fitness chart (Table 3.1) that matches your age and sex.

Table 3.1
Fitness Charts for Men and Women at Various Ages

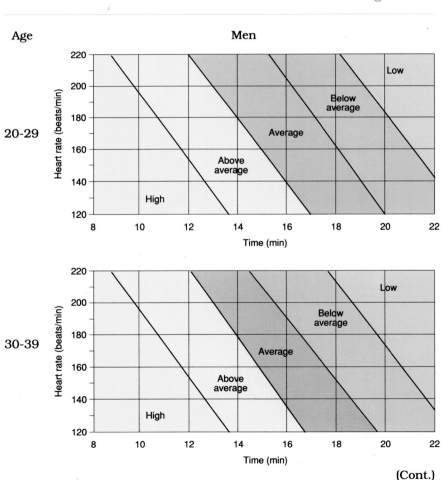

(Cont.)

Table 3.1
(Continued)

Age   Men

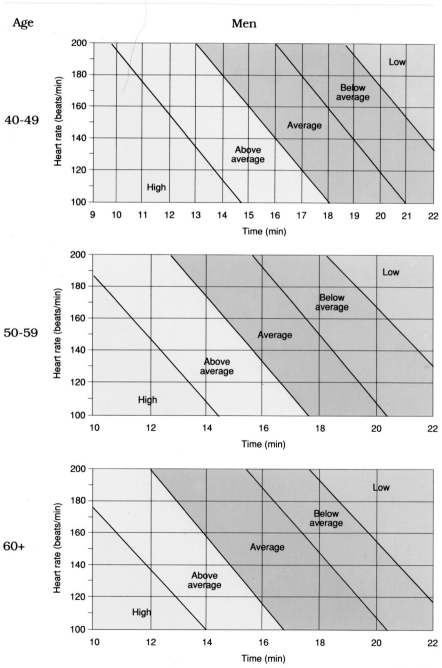

(Cont.)

Table 3.1
(Continued)

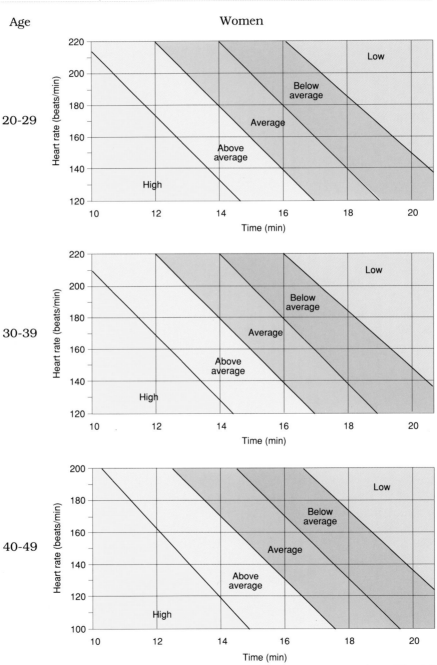

(Cont.)

Table 3.1
(Continued)

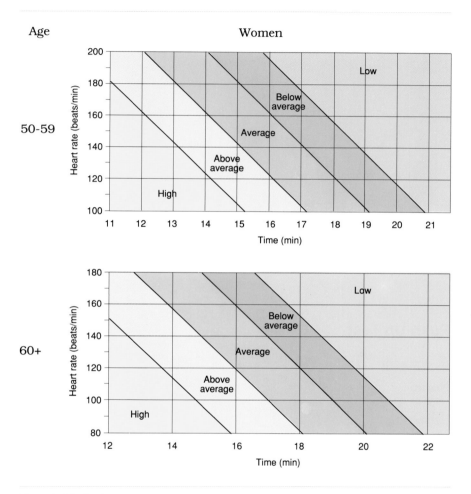

Age   Women

50-59

60+

2. Locate your adjusted one-mile walking time on the horizontal axis and draw a line straight up from that.

3. On the vertical axis, locate your heart rate upon completing the test, and draw a horizontal line to meet the vertical line. That point determines your cardiorespiratory fitness level.

4. Circle the fitness category that corresponds to the area where the lines on your chart intersect. (If you fall

into the High or Above Average categories on the chart, circle High.)

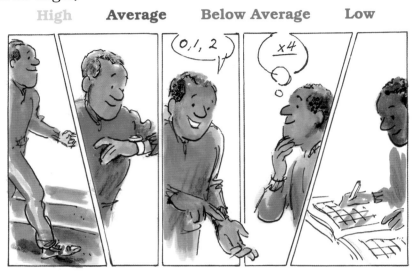

Part II: Muscular Strength and Endurance
Push-Up Test

Equipment:

None

Preparation

Warm up by doing the triceps stretch and shoulder stretch (see page 25). Be sure you know how to perform a push-up correctly (men and women use different techniques, as described here):

- Position yourself on the floor so that your body is straight and your weight is on the hands and feet (men) or hands and knees (women). Be sure your hands are flat on the floor and directly under your shoulders (see Figure 3.2).
- Lower your chest until it touches the floor, then push yourself back up to the starting position. Exhale each time you push your body up; do not hold your breath.
- Keep your body straight, and fully straighten your arms at the end of each push-up.

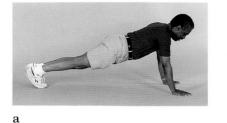
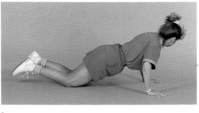

a   b

Figure 3.2   Correct push-up position for (a) men and (b) women.

Procedure

1. Assume the correct position.
2. Begin the first push-up.
3. Count one each time you do a push-up correctly.
4. Stop the test when you must stop to rest.
5. Record the number of push-ups you were able to do.
   _____ push-ups

Results

1. Compare your score to the standards in Table 3.2.

Table 3.2
Muscular Fitness Norms (Push-Ups)

	Score at age				
	20-29	30-39	40-49	50-59	60+
Men					
High	≥ 45	≥ 35	≥ 30	≥ 25	≥ 20
Average	35-44	25-34	20-29	15-24	10-19
Below average	20-34	15-24	12-19	8-14	5-9
Low	< 19	< 14	< 11	< 7	< 4
Women					
High	≥ 34	≥ 25	≥ 20	≥ 15	≥ 5
Average	17-33	12-24	8-19	6-14	3-4
Below average	6-16	4-11	3-7	1-5	1-2
Low	< 5	< 3	< 2	0	0

Note. Adapted by permission of Macmillan Publishing Company from *Health and Fitness Through Physical Activity* by M.L. Pollock, J.H. Wilmore, & S.M. Fox. Copyright © 1978 (New York: Macmillan Publishing Company).

2. Circle your fitness category:

High   **Average**   **Below Average**   **Low**

Part III: Flexibility
Modified Sit-and-Reach Test

Equipment:

Yardstick and adhesive tape

Preparation

1. Place a yardstick on the floor with the zero mark closest to you. Tape the yardstick in place at the 15-inch mark (Figure 3.3).

2. Ask a friend to help you keep your legs straight during the sit-and-reach test. However, it is important that he or she not interfere with your movement.

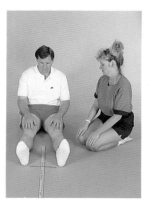

Figure 3.3 The prestretch position for the modified sit-and-reach test.

Procedure

1. Warm up properly using the exercises on page 25.

2. Sit on the floor with the yardstick between your legs, your feet 10 to 12 inches apart, and your heels even with the tape at the 15-inch mark.

3. Place one hand over the other. The tips of your two middle fingers should be on top of one another.

4. Slowly stretch forward *without bouncing or jerking* and slide your fingertips along the yardstick as far as possible (Figure 3.4). The greater your reach, the higher your score will be.

5. Do the test three times.

6. Record your best score to the nearest inch. _____ inches

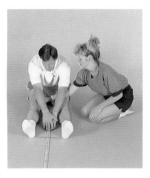

Figure 3.4 The stretched position for the modified sit-and-reach test.

Results

1. Compare your score to the standards in Table 3.3.

Table 3.3
Modified Sit-and-Reach

	Score at age				
	20-29	30-39	40-49	50-59	60+
Men					
High	≥ 19	≥ 18	≥ 17	≥ 16	≥ 15
Average	13-18	12-17	11-16	10-15	9-14
Below average	10-12	9-11	8-10	7-9	6-8
Low	< 9	< 8	< 7	< 6	< 5
Women					
High	≥ 22	≥ 21	≥ 20	≥ 19	≥ 18
Average	16-21	15-20	14-19	13-18	12-17
Below average	13-15	12-14	11-13	10-12	9-11
Low	< 12	< 11	< 10	< 9	< 8

Note. Reprinted by permission from *ACSM Resource Manual for Guidelines for Exercise Testing and Prescription* (p. 165) by S. Blair, P. Painter, R.R. Pate, L.K. Smith, and C.B. Taylor, 1988, Philadelphia: Lea & Febiger, which was adapted from *The Y's Way to Physical Fitness* (pp. 106-111) by L.A. Golding, C.R. Myers, and W.E. Sinning (Eds.), 1982, Rosemont, IL: YMCA of the USA.

2. Circle your fitness category:

High   **Average**   **Below Average**   **Low**

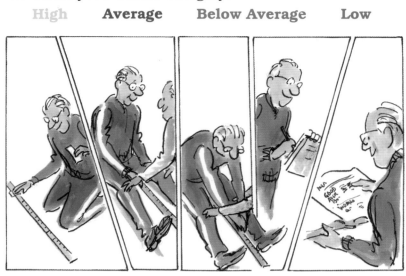

Part IV: Body Composition
Body Mass Index

Equipment:

Body Mass Index chart, a body weight scale, and a ruler

Preparation

1. Wearing minimal clothing and no shoes measure your body weight.

2. Measure your height; to get the most accurate measurement, remove your shoes, stand tall with heels together, and take a deep breath.

Procedure

1. Locate the Body Mass Index chart (Table 3.4) on page 35.

2. Locate your height (in inches) at the top of the scale.

3. Locate your weight (in pounds) on the left side of the scale.

4. Record the fitness category where the two values intersect. _____

Table 3.4

Body Mass Index Chart

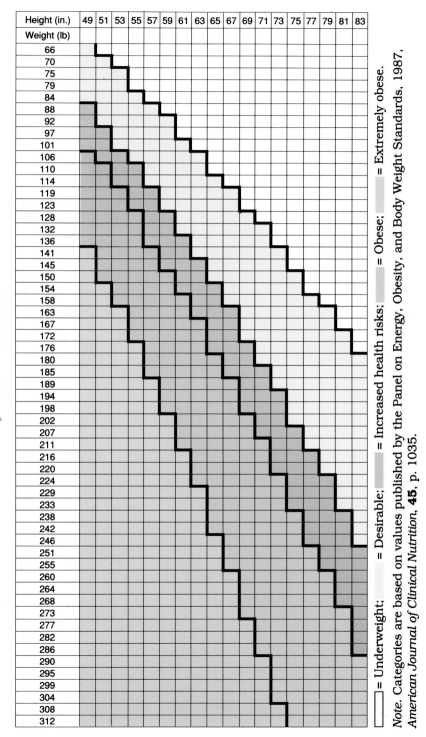

= Underweight;   = Desirable;   = Increased health risks;   = Obese;   = Extremely obese.

Note. Categories are based on values published by the Panel on Energy, Obesity, and Body Weight Standards, 1987, *American Journal of Clinical Nutrition,* **45**, p. 1035.

Result

Circle the appropriate fitness category. (Note that the categories for this score differ from the other three.) Please be aware that there are also health risks associated with being underweight.

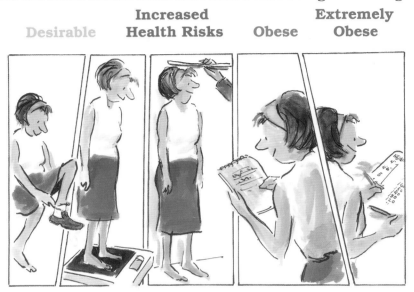

| Desirable | Increased Health Risks | Obese | Extremely Obese |

Physical Fitness Assessment Scorecard

Now that you have taken the four parts of the ACSM Fitness Test, it's time to review your results. Circle your fitness category for each physical fitness component on the Personal Physical Fitness Profile on the next page. Your four scores will give you a clear picture of your individual fitness profile, which will help you build the ACSM Fitness Program most appropriate for you.

Personal Physical Fitness Profile

Component	*Fitness category*			
Cardiorespiratory fitness	High	Average	Below average	Low
Muscular strength and endurance	High	Average	Below average	Low
Flexibility	High	Average	Below average	Low
Body composition	Desirable	Increased health risks	Obese	Extremely obese

Beginning Exercises

T hink back to any previous experiences you've had with exercise. Remember the calisthenics—the jumping jacks, sit-ups, squat thrusts? Do you remember stretching—toe touches, back bends, deep knee bends? Many once-popular exercises have been replaced by safer, more effective alternatives. And it is now widely accepted that exercise does *not* have to hurt to be effective ("No pain, no gain" is just not true!).

This chapter explains how to do the exercises that will become your individualized fitness program.

Cardiorespiratory Endurance

There are many activities that can improve cardiorespiratory endurance. One of the best is walking. Walking can be done almost anywhere and requires no special equipment. Almost anyone can walk for fitness because walking places very little strain on the joints. Walking involves all the major muscle groups, and you can walk at your own pace, alone or with a group. For all of these reasons, walking is one of the most popular forms of exercise.

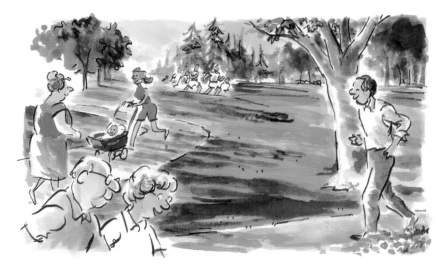

There are some guidelines you should follow when walking for fitness:

- Walk only if you are feeling well. Don't try to exercise through a cold, flu, or other illness. Wait until you are feeling better before resuming your program.
- Remember that walking should leave you feeling invigorated, not exhausted. If you are feeling tired during the day, slow down your workout.
- Wear loose and comfortable exercise clothing.
- Warm up before and cool down after each walking session.
- When you walk in hot weather, take special care:
  —Slow down your walk.
  —Walk in the early morning or evening or in an air-conditioned mall.
  —Drink plenty of water before, during, and after exercise.
  —Cool down for a longer period.

Muscular Strength and Endurance

A high level of muscle strength and endurance will allow your muscles to work longer before they get tired. You can do many different exercises to improve your muscles' ability to work. However, they won't get rid of fat specifically in the area that is being exercised. Despite wishful thinking and advertising claims, reducing fat in a certain spot is not possible. Fat is lost from the entire body, not a specific area. The exercises presented in this section improve muscle strength and endurance; they do not reduce fat.

Some calisthenics that have been popular for years should be avoided by certain exercisers because they could lead to injury, or by everyone simply because they are less effective than other exercises.

Less-Effective Traditional Calisthenics

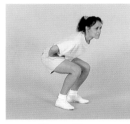

Deep Knee
Bends

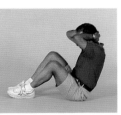

Full Sit-Ups

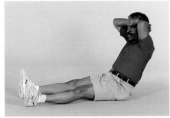

Straight Leg Sit-Ups

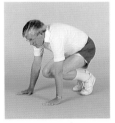

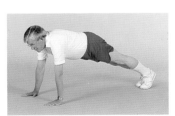

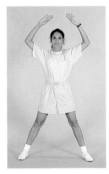

Squat Thrusts
Squat position and thrust position

Jumping
Jacks

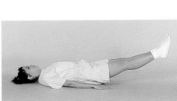

Double Leg Lifts

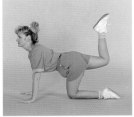

Donkey Kicks

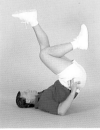

Bicycles

In place of these risky exercises, we recommend you do the safe ones suggested on pages 42 to 50.

ARMS, SHOULDERS, AND CHEST

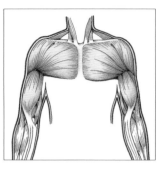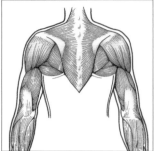

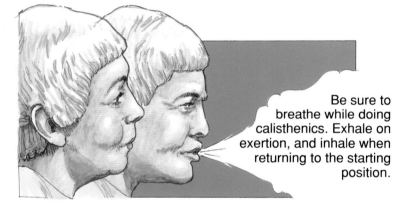

Be sure to breathe while doing calisthenics. Exhale on exertion, and inhale when returning to the starting position.

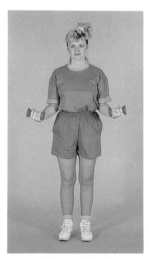

Biceps Curl
Bend at the elbow

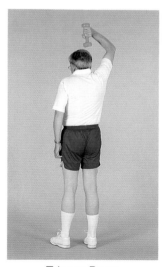

Triceps Press
Keep elbow high; lower and lift weight from behind

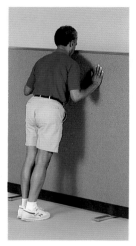

Wall Push-Up
*Push your body away
from the wall*

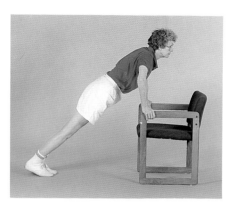

Chair Push-Up
Position chair so it won't slide

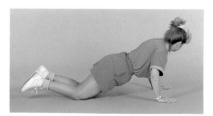

Knee Push-Up
*Keep body straight
from knees to shoulders*

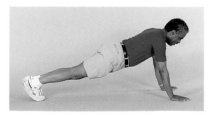

Toe Push-Up
Don't arch your back or lift your hips

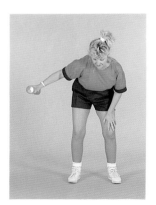

Reverse Fly
*Use shoulder and upper
back muscles to lift weight
to the side and up*

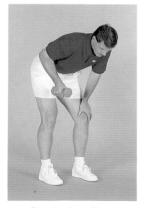

Single Arm Row
*Pull weight to shoulders,
then ease to floor*

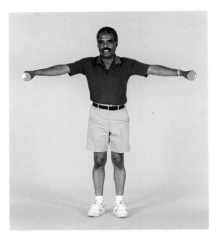

Lateral Raise
Keep elbows slightly bent

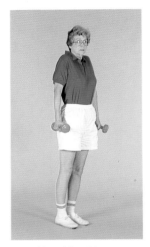

Shoulder Shrug
*Keep arms straight
and lift shoulders
toward ears*

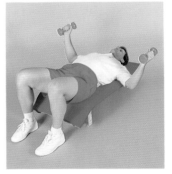

Chest Fly
*Keep elbows slightly bent;
bring both weights high
over chest*

ABDOMINALS

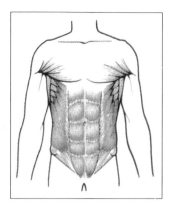

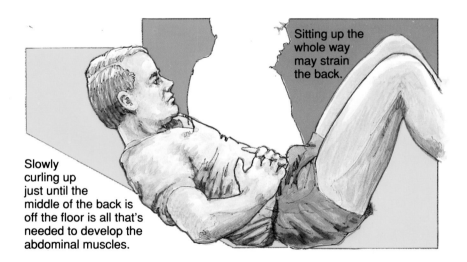

Sitting up the whole way may strain the back.

Slowly curling up just until the middle of the back is off the floor is all that's needed to develop the abdominal muscles.

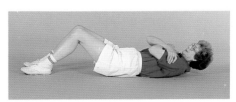

Neck Curl-Up
Only lift head and neck

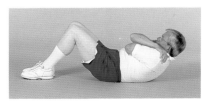

Shoulder Curl-Up
Lift upper back off the floor

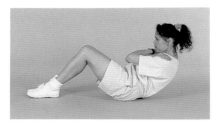

Crossed-Arm Curl-Up
Keep chin slightly tucked

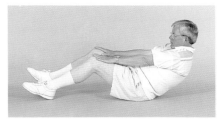

Straight Arm Curl-Up
With Hands on Legs
Slide hands up legs to knees

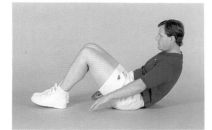

Straight Arm Curl-Up
With Hands on Floor
Slide hands along floor

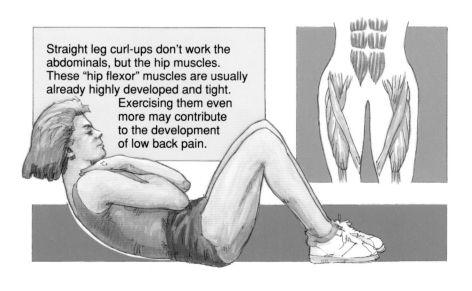

Straight leg curl-ups don't work the abdominals, but the hip muscles. These "hip flexor" muscles are usually already highly developed and tight. Exercising them even more may contribute to the development of low back pain.

GLUTEALS AND HAMSTRINGS

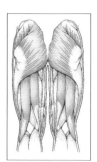

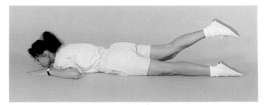

Hamstring Curl
You may want to use ankle weights

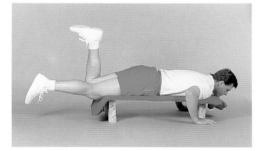

Leg Lift
Lift the whole leg from the hip

HIP ABDUCTORS AND ADDUCTORS

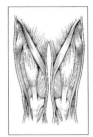

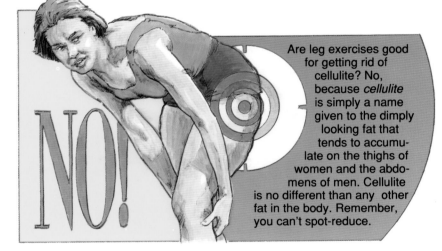

Are leg exercises good for getting rid of cellulite? No, because *cellulite* is simply a name given to the dimply looking fat that tends to accumulate on the thighs of women and the abdomens of men. Cellulite is no different than any other fat in the body. Remember, you can't spot-reduce.

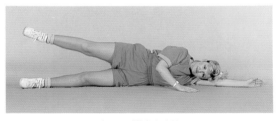

Outer Thigh Lift
Slowly lift and lower upper leg

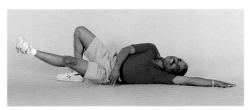

Inner Thigh Lift
Lift lower leg off the floor

QUADRICEPS

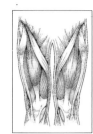

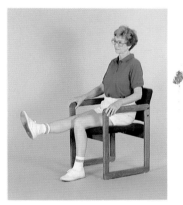

Seated Lower Leg Lift
Lift foot off the floor

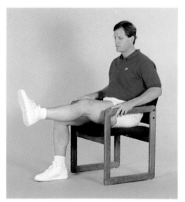

Seated Straight Leg Lift
Raise entire leg off the chair

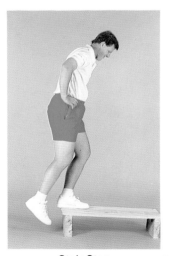

Stair Step
*Step first with right leg
leading, then with left*

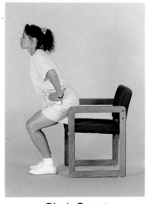

Chair Squat
Do not arch the back

LOWER BACK

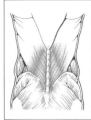

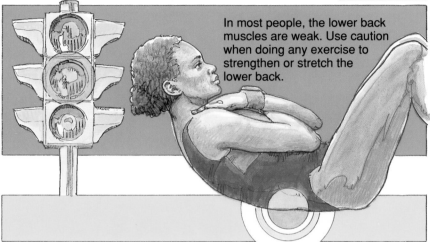

In most people, the lower back muscles are weak. Use caution when doing any exercise to strengthen or stretch the lower back.

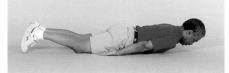

Prone Neck Lift
Avoid arching your neck backward

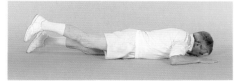

Prone Single Leg Lift
Lift the entire leg from the hip

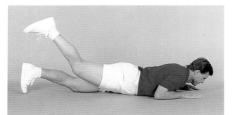

Prone Head and Leg Lift
Lift head and leg at the same time

Some of these recommended calisthenics can also be done with hand or leg weights. When using hand weights, be sure to start with very low weight, and increase weight gradually. Make all movements slowly. If weights cause pain in a joint, stop using them.

Every muscle group can also be worked in a weight room with a variety of weight training equipment. Be sure to have a qualified person show you how to use the equipment safely.

Many women think they should avoid exercising with weights because they don't want to develop large muscles. For most women that can't happen; their genetic makeup prohibits their muscles from growing as large as most men's.

If you want to increase the intensity of your workout but don't have access to weight training equipment, use plastic milk or detergent jugs with easy-grip handles. Partially fill the jugs with water or sand. As you get stronger you can add more water or sand to increase the weight.

Whatever equipment or weight you might use, what is most important is that you do the exercises safely and correctly in order to get the most out of your program.

Remember these tips when you do calisthenics:

- Do all movements in a slow, controlled fashion.
- Maintain normal breathing throughout the movement.
- Stop any exercise that causes pain.
- Stretch each muscle group after your workout.

Stretching: The Safe Way to Improve Flexibility

Remember that flexibility is the ability to move your joints freely and without pain through a wide range of motion. This ability requires that the muscles around the joints be stretched regularly. Every group of muscles in the body can be stretched safely without causing injury to your joints. A safe stretch is one that is *gentle* and *relaxing*; you move just until you can feel the muscle stretch. Hold the position for 10 to 20 seconds, relax, and repeat 3 to 5 times. If a stretch hurts, stop doing it. Pain is a signal from your body that something is wrong. Listen to your body!

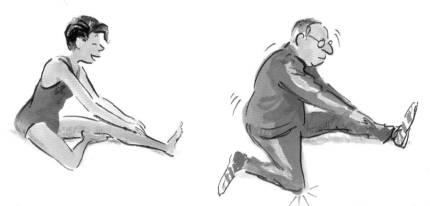

Certain very common stretching exercises should be avoided by some exercisers because they may lead to injury.

Less-Effective Common Stretches

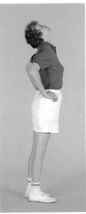

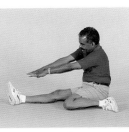

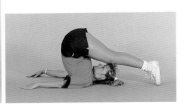

| Standing Toe Touch | Hurdler Stretch | The Plow |

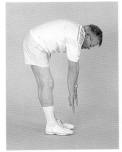

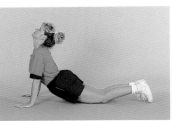

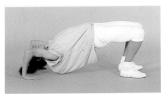

Full Neck Circles   Cobra—Back Hyperextension in Prone Position   Back Bends

Safe, effective exercises for stretching each group of muscles in the body are on pages 53-60.

NECK

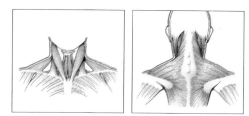

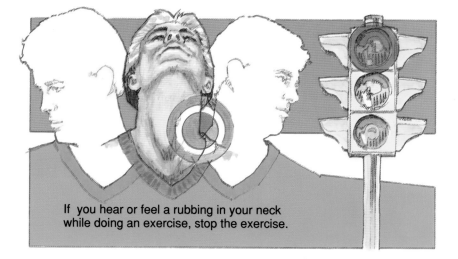

If you hear or feel a rubbing in your neck while doing an exercise, stop the exercise.

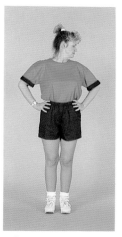

Side to Side Look
Turn head slowly

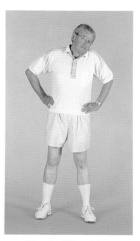

Ear to Shoulder
Keep shoulders relaxed

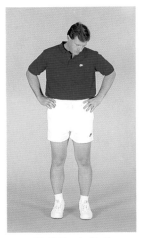

Half Neck Roll
Turn head slowly

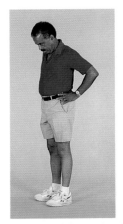

Forward and Down Look
Don't put chin on chest

SHOULDER, CHEST, AND UPPER BACK

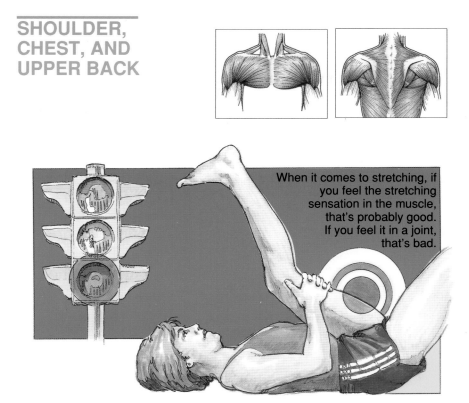

When it comes to stretching, if you feel the stretching sensation in the muscle, that's probably good. If you feel it in a joint, that's bad.

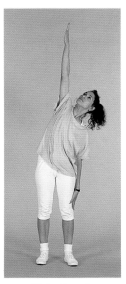

Side Reach
Reach up, not over

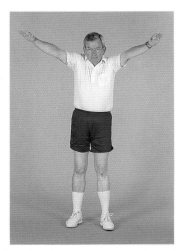

Arm Circle (forward or backward)
Circle arms slowly from shoulder

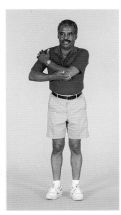

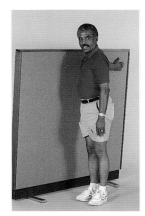

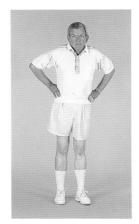

Shoulder Stretch
*Use hand to hold arm,
not to push on elbow*

Chest Stretch
Use a wall

Shoulder Roll
(forward or backward)
*Rotate shoulders only;
leave hands on hips*

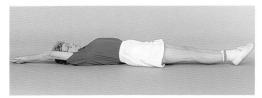

Whole Body Stretch
Keep lower back flat on the floor

LOWER BACK, ABDOMINALS, AND HAMSTRINGS

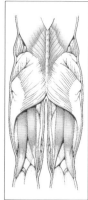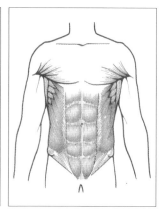

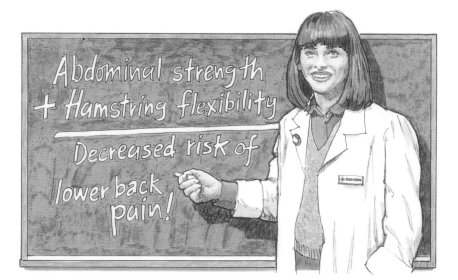

Abdominal strength + Hamstring flexibility

Decreased risk of lower back pain!

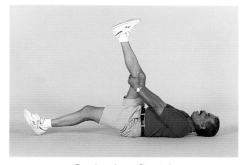

Supine Leg Stretch
Keep leg bent

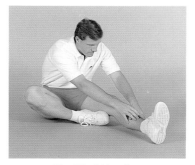

Modified Hurdler
Place foot on inside of straight leg

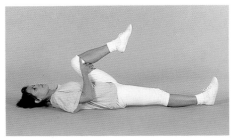
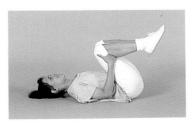

Knee to Chest
One knee at a time, then both; hands under thighs

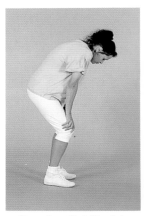
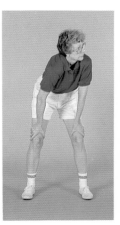
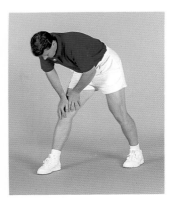

Standing Cat Stretch
Don't arch the back when returning from curled position

Shoulder Turn
Keep knees bent

Standing Hamstring Stretch
Keep knees slightly bent

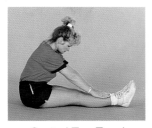
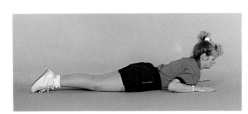

Seated Toe Touch
Don't lock knees

Elbow Cobra
Keep abdomen on floor

INNER THIGH, QUADRICEPS, AND HIP MUSCLES

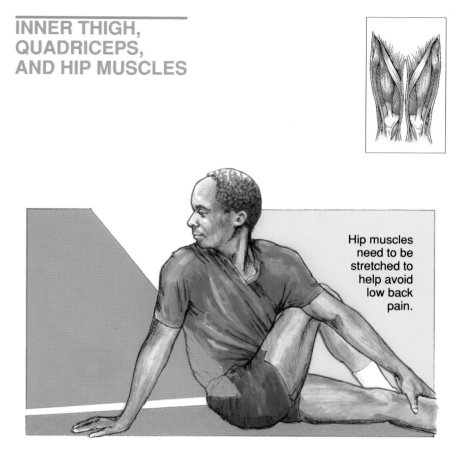

Hip muscles need to be stretched to help avoid low back pain.

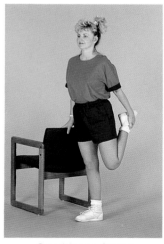

Quadriceps Stretch
Bring foot back toward gluteals

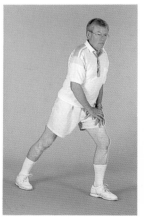

Standing Lunge
Keep knee in line with toe

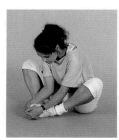

Butterfly
Lean forward gently

GLUTEALS

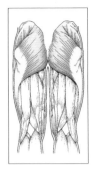

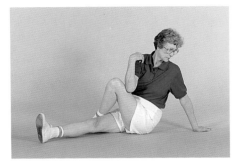

Seated Stretch
*Elbow pushes knee one way
while upper body turns the other*

CALVES

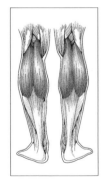

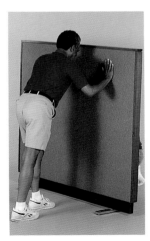

Wall Lean
*Keep back heel on
ground and foot turned
slightly inward*

Stretching should be a pleasant, relaxing part of your exercise program. Remember to listen to your body when doing these stretches, and avoid any exercise that causes pain to your joints.

Body Composition

Aerobic exercise can help change the portion of your body weight that is made up of fat. The best type of exercise for decreasing your body fat is low-to-moderate intensity aerobic exercise—like walking!

Exercise also increases the portion of your body weight that is made up of muscle. The exercises for muscular strength and endurance explained earlier in this chapter will help to increase your muscle.

IIII *Chapter 5*

The ACSM Fitness Program

$\mathbf{T}$his chapter presents the color-coded activity plans with which you will create your personal exercise program, so you can exercise at your own level in every area of fitness.

Using Your Color-Coded ACSM Fitness Program

Look back at page 37, where you recorded your results on the ACSM Fitness Test and then prepared a personal physical fitness profile. Note that the fitness levels are designated by colors:

■ Low	= Level 1	▬▬▬▬▬▬▬▬▬
■ Below average	= Level 2	▬▬▬▬▬▬▬▬▬
■ Average	= Level 3	▬▬▬▬▬▬▬▬▬
■ High	= Level 4	▬▬▬▬▬▬▬▬▬

In circling your fitness levels for cardiorespiratory fitness, muscular strength and endurance, and flexibility, you identified the color-coded programs that you'll be using for each of these three fitness components. Whether you're at the same level or different ones for each component, with the ACSM Fitness Program your exercise is suited to *your* individual fitness. (You also assessed your body composition, and we'll use your walking programs to help you attain or maintain a healthy body composition.)

Now, let's assemble your ACSM Fitness Program.

1. On pages 69 to 72, you'll find four color-coded exercise programs for warming up and building cardiorespiratory fitness. Mark the page on which the program that matches the level of your cardiorespiratory fitness assessment appears (refer to your personal physical fitness profile on page 37).

2. On pages 73 to 76 are the four color-coded exercise programs for muscular strength and endurance. Mark the page on which the program that matches the level of your muscular endurance assessment appears (refer to your profile on page 37).

3. Finally, you'll find the four color-coded flexibility exercise programs on pages 77 to 80. Mark the page on which the program that matches the level of your flexibility assessment appears (refer to your profile on page 37).

By combining the three sets of exercises you've just identified, you have created a complete and personalized program of exercise designed to help you develop your personal fitness.

Each exercise program lists the pages where the exercises are explained in chapter 4. Carefully read the descriptions of all exercises to ensure that you do them safely and effectively (you may need to review them several times when you first begin your program). Any basic equipment you might need to complete your exercises is listed.

Your personal version of the ACSM Fitness Program provides activities to enhance every area of physical fitness. You should complete all of the exercises in the sequence given, but if you experience any pain when doing an exercise, stop that exercise and go on to the next. During your next exercise session, try all of the exercises again. If you still have pain while doing a particular exercise, eliminate it from your program. However, a day or two after you begin an exercise program, you may feel a bit stiff; this is normal and the soreness should disappear in a few days.

The exercise program should be done at least 3 days each week, but no more than 5. Your body responds best to an exercise program if it gets periodic rest. If improving body composition is one of your fitness goals, exercise 5 days a week. If you choose to exercise 3 or 4 days, it's best to leave one day of rest between exercise sessions.

On pages 81 to 92 are exercise logs on which you can record your progress for the 6 weeks of the program. Each time you exercise, record the date at the top of a new column of the exercise log. Check off all exercises you completed. Don't go on to the next level in any particular exercise until you can complete the number or time listed. You may continue to progress in the other exercises, even if you must stay back in a particular exercise for several days. This way, you'll be able to tailor your exercise program to your specific fitness level.

Note in the appropriate space on the exercise log how you felt as you performed the exercises during the week. Be sure to save all of your completed sheets as a record of your progress. When you finish your 6 weeks, continue with all exercises in the program until any slower-moving exercises have caught up.

Eating and Drinking for Action

Proper nutrition is important to any good fitness program. The following points address questions you may have about how your fitness program affects your nutritional needs.

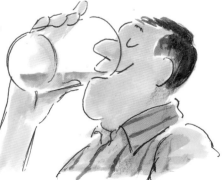

• You need extra water with exercise. Drink a cup of water 15 to 30 minutes before you exercise. And if the weather is hot or the exercise area overly warm, stop for water every 15 to 20 minutes while you're exercising. Drink extra water throughout the day as well.

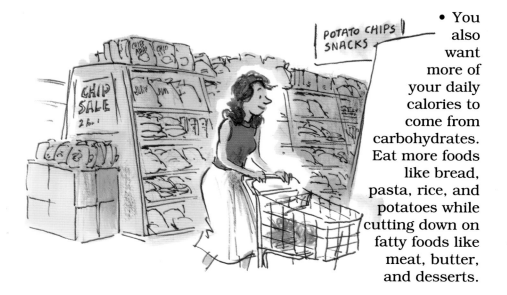

• You also want more of your daily calories to come from carbohydrates. Eat more foods like bread, pasta, rice, and potatoes while cutting down on fatty foods like meat, butter, and desserts.

• You don't need any extra vitamins just because you've started an exercise program.

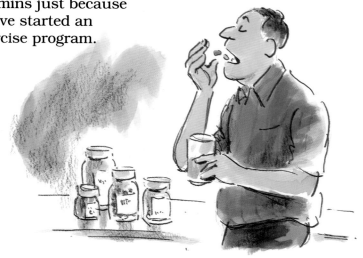

- If you are on a medically supervised diet, you can still do these exercises safely—they will increase your weight loss in addition to building your fitness.

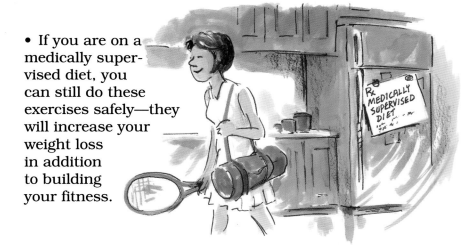

When You've Completed Your Color-Coded Program

Congratulations! You deserve to feel very good about yourself. You've made an important decision, done some work, and progressed toward your goals. You've proven to yourself that *you* can take charge of your exercise habits. Now for the next step.

First, evaluate your progress and your goals. Begin by retaking the ACSM Fitness Test in chapter 3. Are you satisfied with your fitness level? Would you like to continue to increase it? Do you want to keep exercising without changing the intensity of your exercise? Review your reasons for exercising as you listed them on pages 2 and 3. Are they the same now? Next, reexamine your goals (refer to page 15). Have you met your goals? Do you want to set new ones? Your answers to these questions will help lead you to your next step.

If you're satisfied with your progress and your fitness, continue with the Week 6 exercises of your individual program. Perhaps you want to add some variety without really increasing exercise intensity. Chapter 6 provides some alternative exercise methods that can add interest and increase your enjoyment of your exercise program.

If you would like to continue to increase your fitness level, and if your scores on the fitness reevaluation indicate that you are ready for a different exercise program in any area, you can move to the next level of the color-coded program (from Level 1 to Level 2, Level 2 to Level 3, or Level 3 to Level 4) for the fitness area selected. If you've completed the Level 4 program and would like to continue to increase your fitness level, you're ready to begin an entirely new exercise program. Chapter 6 provides valuable information on evaluating programs, equipment, and fitness facilities as you plan for your continuing fitness development.

If your fitness reevaluation indicates that you're not quite ready to begin the next program in any areas of fitness development, continue with the Week 6 exercises of the program you're working in for an additional 3 weeks. Then take the ACSM Fitness Test components in those areas again to determine if you're ready to progress to the next level. Remember, fitness takes commitment!

Whichever exercise program you continue to follow, you can be satisfied in the knowledge that *you* are making the choice to continue your exercise habit. Happy exercising!

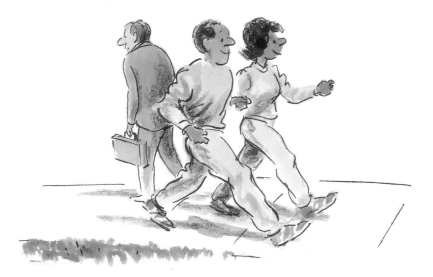

ACSM FITNESS PROGRAMS

Exercises for Warm-Up and Cardiorespiratory Endurance

LEVEL 1

Equipment Needed: Watch or clock with a second hand

	Week					
Exercise	1	2	3	4	5	6
Shoulder Roll (backward) (p. 56)	5x	5x	5x	5x	5x	5x
Forward and Down Look (p. 54)	10 s 2x	10 s 2x	10 s 2x	10 s 2x	10 s 2x	10 s 2x
Walk in Place	2 min	2 min	2 min	2 min	2 min	2 min
Side Reach (alternating sides) (p. 55)	5 ea	5 ea	5 ea	10 ea	10 ea	10 ea
Standing Cat Stretch (p. 58)	10 s 2x	10 s 2x	10 s 2x	10 s 2x	15 s 2x	15 s 2x
Chest Stretch (p. 56)	10 s 1 ea	10 s 1 ea	20 s 1 ea	15 s 1 ea	15 s 1 ea	15 s 1 ea
Wall Lean (p. 60)	10 s 2 ea	10 s 2 ea	10 s 2 ea	15 s 2 ea	15 s 2 ea	15 s 2 ea
Quadriceps Stretch (p. 59)	10 s 1 ea	10 s 1 ea	10 s 1 ea	15 s 1 ea	15 s 1 ea	15 s 1 ea
Walk*	10 min	15 min	15 min	20 min	20 min	20 min

x = times
s = seconds
ea = each side

*Follow these specific guidelines (in minutes) for each week you walk:
    Week 1—5 out, 5 back;
    Week 2—7:30 out, 7:30 back;
    Week 3—8 out, 7 back (you'll have to walk faster on the way back);
    Week 4—10 out, 10 back;
    Week 5—10 out, 10 back; and
    Week 6—10 out, 10 back, and increase distance each day.

LEVEL 2 ▐███████████████████████

Equipment Needed: Watch or clock with a second hand

Week

Exercise	1	2	3	4	5	6
Side to Side Look (p. 53)	5 s 2 ea	5 s 2 ea	5 s 2 ea	5 s 2 ea	5 s 2 ea	5 s 2 ea
Shoulder Roll (backward) (p. 56)	5x	5x	5x	5x	5x	5x
Shoulder Roll (forward) (p. 56)	5x	5x	5x	5x	5x	5x
Walk in Place	2 min	2 min	2 min	2 min	2 min	2 min
Standing Cat Stretch (p. 58)	15 s 2x	15 s 2x	15 s 2x	15 s 2x	15 s 2x	15 s 2x
Knee to Chest (p. 58)	10 s	10 s	10 s	10 s	10 s	10 s
Seated Toe Touch (p. 58)	10 s 2x	10s 2x	10 s 2x	15 s 2x	15 s 2x	15 s 2x
Shoulder Stretch (p. 56)	10 s 1 ea	10 s 1ea	10 s 1ea	15 s 1ea	15 s 1ea	15 s 2 ea
Chest Stretch (p. 56)	10 s 1 ea	10 s 1 ea	10 s 1 ea	15 s 1 ea	15 s 1 ea	15 s 1 ea
Wall Lean (p. 60)	10 s 2 ea	10 s 2 ea	10 s 2 ea	15 s 2 ea	15 s 2 ea	15 s 2 ea
Walk*	20 min	20 min	25 min	25 min	30 min	30 min

x = times
s = seconds
ea = each side

*Follow these specific guidelines (in minutes) for each week you walk:
   Week 1—10 out, 10 back;
   Week 2—10 out, 10 back, and increase distance each day;
   Week 3—12:30 out, 12:30 back;
   Week 4—13 out, 12 back (you'll have to walk faster on the way back);
   Week 5—15 out, 15 back; and
   Week 6—15 out, 15 back, and increase distance each day.

LEVEL 3 ▬▬▬▬▬▬▬▬▬▬▬▬▬▬▬▬

Equipment Needed: Watch or clock with a second hand

	Week					
Exercise	1	2	3	4	5	6
Forward and Down Look (p. 54)	5x	5x	5x	5x	5x	5x
Ear to Shoulder (p. 53)	10 s 2 ea	10 s 2 ea	10 s 2 ea	10 s 2 ea	10 s 2 ea	10 s 2 ea
Walk in Place	2 min	2 min	2 min	2 min	2 min	2 min
Arm Circle (forward) (p. 55) (continue to walk in place)	10x	15x	20x	25x	30x	35x
Arm Circle (backward) (p. 55) (continue to walk in place)	10x	15x	20x	25x	30x	35x
Standing Lunge (p. 59)	10 s 1 ea	10 s 1 ea	10 s 2 ea	10 s 2 ea	10 s 2 ea	10 s 2 ea
Standing Hamstring Stretch (p. 58)	10 s 1 ea	10 s 1 ea	10 s 2 ea	15 s 2 ea	15 s 2 ea	15 s 2 ea
Standing Cat Stretch (p. 58)	15 s 2x	15 s 2x	15 s 2x	15 s 2x	15 s 2x	15 s 2x
Shoulder Turn (p. 58)	10 s 1 ea	10 s 1 ea	10 s 1 ea	15 s 1 ea	15 s 1 ea	15 s 1 ea
Wall Lean (p. 60)	15 s 2 ea	15 s 2 ea	15 s 2 ea	15 s 2 ea	15 s 2 ea	15 s 2 ea
Chest Stretch (p. 56)	15 s 2 ea	15 s 2 ea	15 s 2 ea	15 s 2 ea	15 s 2 ea	15 s 2 ea
Walk*	30 min	30 min	35 min	35 min	40 min	40 min

x = times
s = seconds
ea = each side

*Follow these specific guidelines (in minutes) for each week you walk:
   Week 1—15 out, 15 back;
   Week 2—15 out, 15 back, and increase distance each day;
   Week 3—17:30 out, 17:30 back;
   Week 4—18 out, 17 back (you'll have to walk faster on the way back);
   Week 5—20 out, 20 back; and
   Week 6—20 out, 20 back, and increase distance each day.

LEVEL 4

Equipment Needed: Watch or clock with a second hand

	Week					
Exercise	1	2	3	4	5	6
Shoulder Roll (forward) (p. 56)	10x	10x	10x	10x	10x	10x
Walk (slow pace)	2 min	2 min	2 min	2 min	2 min	2 min
Side Reach (alternating sides) (p.55)	15 s 2 ea	15 s 2 ea	15 s 3 ea	15 s 3 ea	15 s 4 ea	15 s 5 ea
Standing Hamstring Stretch (p. 58)	10 s 1 ea	10 s 2 ea	10 s 2 ea	15 s 2 ea	15 s 2 ea	15 s 2 ea
Wall Lean (p. 60)	10 s 1 ea	10 s 1 ea	10 s 2 ea	15 s 2 ea	15 s 2 ea	15 s 2 ea
Standing Cat Stretch (p. 58)	15 s 2x	15 s 2x	15 s 2x	15 s 2x	15 s 2x	15 s 2x
Shoulder Turn (p. 58)	15 s 2 ea	15 s 2 ea	15 s 3 ea	15 s 3 ea	15 s 3 ea	15 s 3 ea
Quadriceps Stretch (p. 59)	15 s 1 ea	15 s 1 ea	15 s 1 ea	15 s 2 ea	15 s 2 ea	15 s 2 ea
Shoulder Stretch (p. 56)	15 s 2 ea	15 s 2 ea	15 s 2 ea	15 s 2 ea	15 s 2 ea	15 s 2 ea
Chest Stretch (p. 56)	15 s 2 ea	15 s 2 ea	15 s 2 ea	15 s 2 ea	15 s 2 ea	15 s 2 ea
Shoulder Roll (backward) (p. 56)	10x	10x	10x	10x	10x	10x
Ear to Shoulder (p. 53)	5 s 2 ea	5 s 2 ea	5 s 2 ea	5 s 2 ea	5 s 2 ea	5 s 2 ea
Walk*	40 min	40 min	40 min	45 min	45 min	45 min

x = times
s = seconds
ea = each side

*Follow these specific guidelines (in minutes) for each week you walk:
  Week 1—20 out, 20 back;
  Week 2—20 out, 20 back, and increase distance each day;
  Week 3—20:30 out, 19:30 back (you'll have to walk faster on the way back);
  Week 4—22:30 out, 22:30 back;
  Week 5—23 out, 22 back (you'll have to walk faster on the way back); and
  Week 6—try to find an enjoyable loop, rather than an out-and-back path.

Exercises for Muscular Strength and Endurance
LEVEL 1 ▰▰▰▰▰▰▰▰▰▰▰

Equipment Needed

- Plastic jug filled with 1 to 2 pounds of water (2 cups = 1 pound)
- A sturdy chair with arms

			Week			
Exercise	1	2	3	4	5	6
Neck Curl-Up (p. 45)	6	8	10	13	16	20
Wall Push-Up (p. 43)	3	4	6	8	10	12
Single Arm Row (1 to 2 lb) (p. 43)	5 ea	7 ea	9 ea	11 ea	13 ea	15 ea
Seated Lower Leg Lift (p. 49)	—	—	5 ea	6 ea	8 ea	10 ea

x = times
s = seconds
ea = each side

LEVEL 2 ▮▮▮▮▮▮▮▮▮▮▮▮▮▮▮▮▮▮▮▮▮▮▮▮▮▮▮▮▮▮

Equipment Needed

- Plastic jug filled with 3 to 5 pounds of water (2 cups = 1 pound)
- A sturdy chair with arms

Week

Exercise	1	2	3	4	5	6
Shoulder Curl-Up (p. 45)	8	10	12	14	17	20
Chair Push-Up (p. 43)	4	5	6	8	10	12
Single Arm Row (3 to 5 lb) (p. 43)	8 ea	9 ea	10 ea	11 ea	13 ea	15 ea
Seated Straight Leg Lift (p. 49)	10 ea	12 ea	14 ea	16 ea	18 ea	20 ea
Prone Neck Lift (p. 50)	5	6	8	10	12	15

x = times

s = seconds

ea = each side

LEVEL 3

Equipment Needed

- Plastic jug filled with 5 to 8 pounds of water (2 cups = 1 pound)
- A bench or step 10 to 12 inches high

	Week					
Exercise	1	2	3	4	5	6
Straight Arm Curl-Up (p. 46)	8	10	12	14	17	20
Knee Push-Up (p. 43)	8	10	12	14	17	20
Single Arm Row (5 to 8 lb) (p. 43)	8 ea	9 ea	10 ea	11 ea	13 ea	15 ea
Stair Step (10 to 12 in.) (p. 49)	10 ea	12 ea	14 ea	16 ea	18 ea	20 ea
Prone Single Leg Lift (p. 50)	5 ea	6 ea	8 ea	10 ea	12 ea	15 ea

x = times
s = seconds
ea = each side

LEVEL 4

Equipment Needed

- Two plastic jugs, one filled with 2 to 5 pounds of water, the other with 5 to 8 pounds
  (2 cups = 1 pound)
- A sturdy chair with arms

Exercise	Week 1	2	3	4	5	6
Crossed-Arm Curl-Up (p. 46)	10	12	14	16	18	20
Toe Push-Up (p. 43)	4	5	7	9	12	15
Biceps Curl (5 to 8 lb) (p. 42)	5 ea	7 ea	9 ea	11 ea	13 ea	15 ea
Reverse Fly (2 to 5 lb) (p. 43)	5 ea	7 ea	9 ea	11 ea	13 ea	15 ea
Chair Squat (p. 49)	10	12	14	16	18	20
Prone Head and Leg Lift (p. 50)	5 ea	6 ea	8 ea	10 ea	12 ea	15 ea

x = times
s = seconds
ea = each side

Exercises for Flexibility

LEVEL 1 ▆▆▆▆▆▆▆▆▆▆▆▆▆▆▆▆▆▆

Equipment Needed: Watch or clock with a second hand

	Week					
Exercise	1	2	3	4*	5*	6*
Wall Lean (p. 60)	10 s 3 ea	10 s 3 ea	10 s 3 ea	20 s 3 ea	20 s 3 ea	20 s 3 ea
Chest Stretch (p. 56)	10 s 3 ea	10 s 3 ea	10 s 3 ea	20 s 3 ea	20 s 3 ea	20 s 3 ea
Quadriceps Stretch (p. 59)	10 s 3 ea	10 s 3 ea	10 s 3 ea	20 s 3 ea	20 s 3 ea	20 s 3 ea
Seated Toe Touch (p. 58)	10 s 3x	10 s 3x	10 s 3x	20 s 3x	20 s 3x	20 s 3x
Whole Body Stretch (p. 56)	20 s	20 s	20 s	20 s	20 s	20 s

x = times

s = seconds

ea = each side

*When doing these stretches, hold for 10 s, then move a tiny bit further and hold 10 s more.

LEVEL 2 ▌████████████████████████████████

Equipment Needed: Watch or clock with a second hand

Week

Exercise	1	2*	3*	4*	5*	6*
Wall Lean (p. 60)	10 s 3 ea	20 s 3 ea	20 s 3 ea	20 s 3 ea	20 s 3 ea	20 s 3 ea
Chest Stretch (p. 56)	10 s 3 ea	20 s 3 ea	20 s 3 ea	20 s 3 ea	20 s 3 ea	20 s 3 ea
Quadriceps Stretch (p. 59)	10 s 3 ea	20 s 3 ea	20 s 3 ea	20 s 3 ea	20 s 3 ea	20 s 3 ea
Seated Toe Touch (p. 58)	10 s 3x	20 s 3x	20 s 3x	20 s 3x	20 s 3x	20 s 3x
Knee to Chest (p. 58)	10 s 3x	20 s 3x	20 s 3x	20 s 3x	20 s 3x	20 s 3x

x = times
s = seconds
ea = each side

*When doing these stretches, hold for 10 s, then move a tiny bit further and hold 10 s more.

LEVEL 3 ▰▰▰▰▰▰▰▰▰▰▰▰▰▰▰▰

Equipment Needed: Watch or clock with a second hand

Week

Exercise	1	2*	3*	4*	5*	6*
Wall Lean (p. 60)	10 s 3 ea	20 s 3 ea	20 s 3 ea	20 s 3 ea	20 s 3 ea	20 s 3 ea
Chest Stretch (p. 56)	10 s 3 ea	20 s 3 ea	20 s 3 ea	20 s 3 ea	20 s 3 ea	20 s 3 ea
Quadriceps Stretch (p. 59)	10 s 3 ea	20 s 3 ea	20 s 3 ea	20 s 3 ea	20 s 3 ea	20 s 3 ea
Seated Toe Touch (p. 58)	10 s 3x	20 s 3x	20 s 3x	20 s 3x	20 s 3x	20 s 3x
Knee to Chest (both at once) (p. 58)	10 s 3 ea	20 s 3 ea	20 s 3 ea	20 s 3 ea	20 s 3 ea	20 s 3 ea

x = times
s = seconds
ea = each side

*When doing these stretches, hold for 10 s, then move a tiny bit further and hold 10 s more.

LEVEL 4

Equipment Needed: Watch or clock with a second hand

Week

Exercise	1	2*	3*	4*	5*	6*
Wall Lean (p. 60)	10 s 3 ea	20 s 3 ea	20 s 3 ea	20 s 3 ea	20 s 3 ea	20 s 3 ea
Chest Stretch (p. 56)	10 s 3 ea	20 s 3 ea	20 s 3 ea	20 s 3 ea	20 s 3 ea	20 s 3 ea
Quadriceps Stretch (p. 59)	10 s 3 ea	20 s 3 ea	20 s 3 ea	20 s 3 ea	20 s 3 ea	20 s 3 ea
Seated Toe Touch (p. 58)	10 s 3x	20 s 3x	20 s 3x	20 s 3x	20 s 3x	20 s 3x
Knee to Chest (both at once) (p. 58)	10 s 3 ea	20 s 3 ea	20 s 3 ea	20 s 3 ea	20 s 3 ea	20 s 3 ea

x = times

s = seconds

ea = each side

*When doing these stretches, hold for 10 s, then move a tiny bit further and hold 10 s more.

Level 1 Program

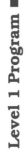

Date	Week 1	Week 2	Week 3	Week 4	Week 5	Week 6
Warm-Up and Cardiorespiratory Endurance						
Shoulder Roll (backward)						
Forward and Down Look						
Walk in Place						
Side Reach (alternating sides)						
Standing Cat Stretch						
Chest Stretch						
Wall Lean						
Quadriceps Stretch						
Walk						

Notes

Level 2 Program

Warm-Up and Cardiorespiratory Endurance	Week 1	Week 2	Week 3	Week 4	Week 5	Week 6
Date						
Side to Side Look						
Shoulder Roll (backward)						
Shoulder Roll (forward)						
Walk in Place						
Standing Cat Stretch						
Knee to Chest						
Seated Toe Touch						
Shoulder Stretch						
Chest Stretch						
Wall Lean						
Walk						
Notes						

Level 3 Program

	Date	Week 1	Week 2	Week 3	Week 4	Week 5	Week 6
Warm-Up and Cardiorespiratory Endurance							
Forward and Down Look							
Ear to Shoulder							
Walk in Place							
Arm Circle (forward)							
Arm Circle (backward)							
Standing Lunge							
Standing Hamstring Stretch							
Standing Cat Stretch							
Shoulder Turn							
Wall Lean							
Chest Stretch							
Walk							
Notes							

Level 4 Program

Warm-Up and Cardiorespiratory Endurance

	Date	Week 1	Week 2	Week 3	Week 4	Week 5	Week 6
Shoulder Roll (forward)							
Walk (slow pace)							
Side Reach (alternating sides)							
Standing Hamstring Stretch							
Wall Lean							
Standing Cat Stretch							
Shoulder Turn							
Quadriceps Stretch							
Shoulder Stretch							
Chest Stretch							
Shoulder Roll (backward)							
Ear to Shoulder							
Walk							
Notes							

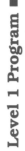

Level 1 Program

	Week 1	Week 2	Week 3	Week 4	Week 5	Week 6
Date						
Muscular Strength and Endurance						
Neck Curl-Up						
Wall Push-Up						
Single Arm Row						
Seated Lower Leg Lift						
Notes						

Level 2 Program

Muscular Strength and Endurance	Date	Week 1	Week 2	Week 3	Week 4	Week 5	Week 6
Shoulder Curl-Up							
Chair Push-Up							
Single Arm Row							
Seated Straight Leg Lift							
Prone Neck Lift							
Notes							

Level 3 Program

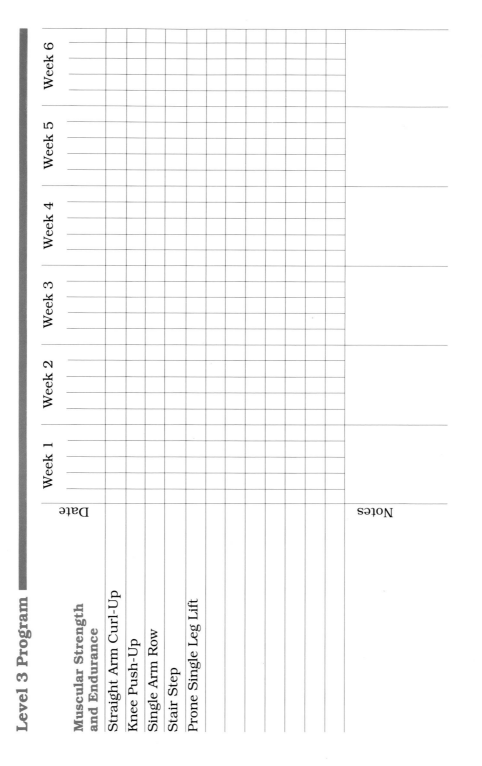

Muscular Strength and Endurance	Week 1	Week 2	Week 3	Week 4	Week 5	Week 6
Date						
Straight Arm Curl-Up						
Knee Push-Up						
Single Arm Row						
Stair Step						
Prone Single Leg Lift						
Notes						

Level 4 Program

Muscular Strength and Endurance

	Week 1	Week 2	Week 3	Week 4	Week 5	Week 6
Date						
Crossed-Arm Curl-Up						
Toe Push-Up						
Biceps Curl						
Reverse Fly						
Chair Squat						
Prone Head and Leg Lift						
Notes						

Level 1 Program

	Week 1	Week 2	Week 3	Week 4	Week 5	Week 6
Date						
Flexibility						
Wall Lean						
Chest Stretch						
Quadriceps Stretch						
Seated Toe Touch						
Whole Body Stretch						
Notes						

Level 2 Program

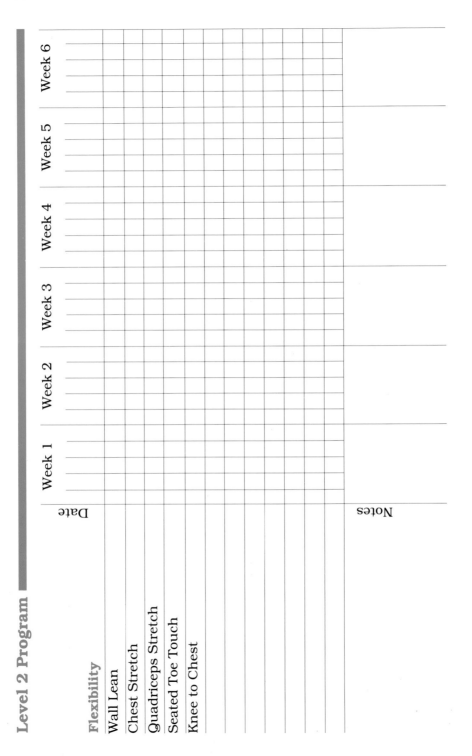

Date	Week 1	Week 2	Week 3	Week 4	Week 5	Week 6
Flexibility						
Wall Lean						
Chest Stretch						
Quadriceps Stretch						
Seated Toe Touch						
Knee to Chest						

Notes

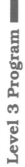

Level 3 Program

Flexibility	Date	Week 1	Week 2	Week 3	Week 4	Week 5	Week 6
Wall Lean							
Chest Stretch							
Quadriceps Stretch							
Seated Toe Touch							
Knees to Chest							

Notes

Level 4 Program

Flexibility

	Date	Week 1	Week 2	Week 3	Week 4	Week 5	Week 6
Wall Lean							
Chest Stretch							
Quadriceps Stretch							
Seated Toe Touch							
Knees to Chest							
Notes							

The Next Step

Congratulations on completing your ACSM Fitness Program! Are you ready for the next step? Do you want to add new activities to your fitness program? Are you interested in joining a fitness center? Are you looking for more information about health and fitness? This chapter has information to help you take that next step.

Choosing Other Aerobic Activities

Walking is not the only exercise that will improve your physical fitness. Other aerobic activities—which use large muscle groups, are rhythmic, and can be done continuously—will give you similar benefits. Such activities include these:

Bicycling	Rope skipping
Cross-country skiing	Rowing
Dancing	Skating
Hiking	Stair climbing
Jogging	Swimming

You can do any of these activities, or a mixture of them, throughout the week. What's important is to do some form of aerobic activity at least 3 days a week.

Guidelines for Aerobic Activity Programs

Regardless of which aerobic activities you do, follow these guidelines to improve your fitness:

- Exercise 3 to 5 days each week.
- Warm-up for 5 to 10 minutes before each aerobic activity session.
- Maintain your desired exercise intensity for 20 to 60 minutes.
- Gradually decrease your activity to cool down, and stretch for 5 to 10 minutes.

If weight loss is the main reason you are exercising, do aerobic activity for at least 30 minutes 5 days a week.

What to Look for in Aerobic Activity

There are several factors to consider when adding other aerobic activities to your fitness program:

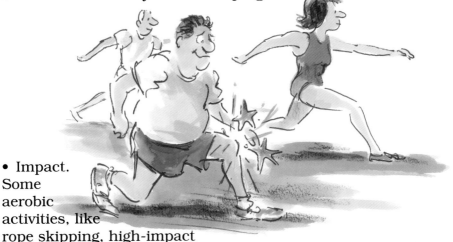

- Impact. Some aerobic activities, like rope skipping, high-impact aerobics, and running, involve jumping and pounding that becomes uncomfortable for some people when done too long or too often. Swimming, cross-country skiing, cycling, rowing, and hiking are "low-impact" and easier on the joints.

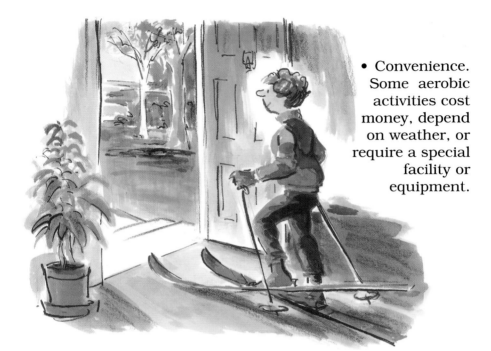

• Convenience. Some aerobic activities cost money, depend on weather, or require a special facility or equipment.

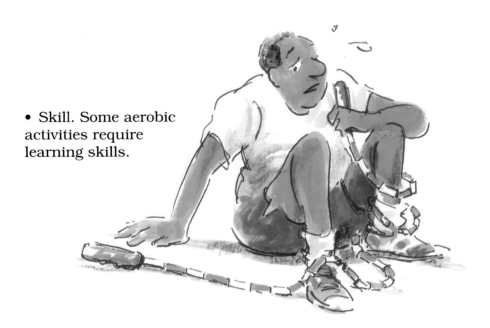

• Skill. Some aerobic activities require learning skills.

• Social factors. Most aerobic activities can be done alone or with a group. Sometimes exercising with a group is more fun.

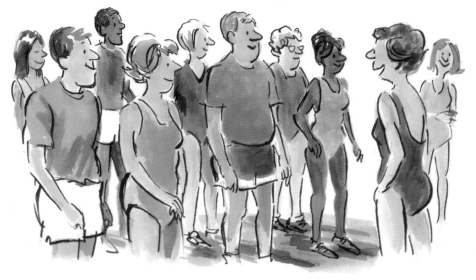

• Enjoyment. By finding an activity you enjoy you're more likely to stick with it. Including several activities in your fitness program helps prevent boredom.

Finding the Right Intensity

One way to tell if your intensity is a good one is by checking your heart rate. Determine your target heart rate range using the steps described in the box. Then during your aerobic activity find your pulse at one of the places shown in chapter 3 (see page 24). If your beats per minute are within your target heart rate range, your pace is good.

Determining Your Target Heart Rate

1. Calculate your approximate maximum heart rate:

   220 – age = _____ (maximum heart rate)

2. Multiply your approximate maximum heart rate by 0.6:

   Maximum heart rate x 0.6 = _____

   This number is your lower heart rate limit for aerobic exercise.

3. Multiply your maximum heart rate by 0.8:

   Maximum heart rate x 0.8 = _____

   This number is your upper limit heart rate for aerobic exercise.

4. Your target heart rate range during aerobic exercise, then, is defined by your lower and upper heart rate limits.

Caution: If you take heart or blood pressure medication, your range during exercise may be lower than these calculations; see your physician before using this target heart rate range.

By reaching and maintaining a heart rate in your target range during aerobic activity for 20 to 60 minutes 3 to 5 days each week, you can be sure of experiencing the physical and mental benefits of exercise.

Exercising at a low to moderate pace for a longer time is better than exercising at a high pace for a short time. Why?

- There is less risk of orthopedic problems occurring.
- You are less likely to suffer injuries.
- You are more likely to stay with your exercise program.
- You can still improve your level of fitness.

Increasing Daily Physical Activity

It is important to your health that, in addition to your regular aerobic activity, you are physically active every day. You can increase your daily physical activity in many ways:

- Walk to do short errands instead of driving.
- When you drive, park some distance from your destination.
- Take stairs instead of elevators and escalators.
- Do your own lawn work (try a push mower rather than a garden tractor), gardening, and housework.
- During coffee breaks at work, take a short walk.
- Walk on the golf course instead of taking a cart.

And on days when you don't have time for your entire workout, do whatever you can, even if it's just 10 to 15 minutes of your program. Don't skip an entire workout just because you can't complete it. Remember, all appropriate physical activity contributes to health!

Continuing Muscular Endurance Activity

In addition to aerobic activity, you should also continue muscular strength and endurance activities. You can keep doing the exercises described in chapter 3 (using jugs or hand or wrist weights), or you may want to join a fitness center or purchase home weight training equipment. Follow these simple guidelines to be sure that you're getting the most out of your program:

Guidelines for Muscular Strength and Endurance Programs

- Your workout should consist of 8 to 10 exercises that use the major muscle groups shown in chapter 3.
- You should do 8 to 12 repetitions of each exercise.
- Once you can do 12 repetitions of an exercise you are ready to move on. During your next exercise session you should either increase the weight used or use the same amount of weight and do 12 repetitions of the exercise, rest briefly, then do another 8 to 12 repetitions of the same exercise.

Missing a workout occasionally will not affect your fitness. However, after missing workouts for 2 weeks, you may begin to see a decline in fitness level. After 3 to 5 months of not working out, you may have lost all the ground you had gained since beginning to work out.

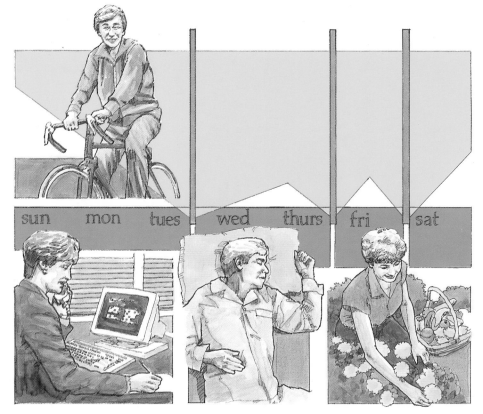

sun   mon   tues   wed   thurs   fri   sat

Trying Something Different

If you are ready for some variety, there are many options available. Most communities have fitness centers, and stores are filled with exercise equipment and videos and fitness books. Community recreation programs also offer fitness programs. How do you decide what is right for you?

Choosing Home Exercise Equipment

You may choose to expand your exercise program at home by purchasing aerobic or weight training equipment. Exercising at home saves both time and the expense of fitness club membership; it also allows you to exercise in privacy.

There are many different types of exercise equipment on the market. Choices can range from $20 collapsible equipment to $10,000 state-of-the-art models. How do you choose what is right for you?

Not every piece of exercise equipment for sale in stores, through magazines, or on television will produce desired results. If an advertiser's claim seems too good to be true, then it probably is! If possible, you should try out any equipment before you buy it.

Products You Should Avoid

- Those that claim you'll see results immediately

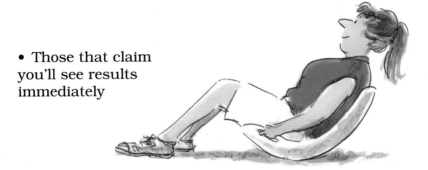

- Those that claim to make exercise an effortless, no-sweat workout

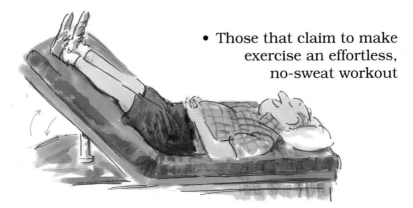

• Those that claim to
remove fat from a certain
area or to get rid
of "cellulite"

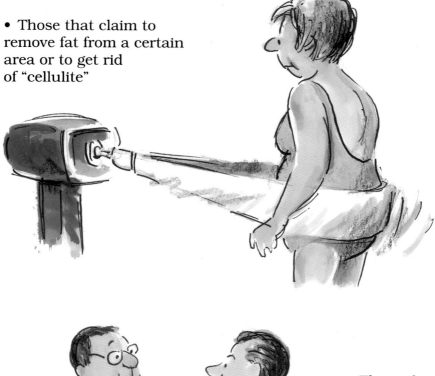

• Those that
claim that
wearing
special
equipment
or clothing
while
exercising
will help you
lose weight

Choosing a Fitness Center

Some people find home exercise lonely or boring and want the variety and socializing that a fitness center can offer. Just as with home exercise equipment, you need to evaluate and compare fitness centers before joining one. Centers vary in what they offer, what they cost, and what quality they provide. Visit each center at the time of day you intend to use it. Try out equipment and talk to the staff.

Choosing a Fitness Book or Video

It seems every entertainment celebrity has a fitness product on the market. Preview videos and examine books carefully before you buy.

Use the checklists that follow to help you decide which aerobic or weight training equipment, fitness center, or fitness book or video is right for you.

Choosing Cardiorespiratory Exercise Equipment

Take this checklist to the store with you. Compare several models; put a check next to questions that you can answer "yes." The model with the most checks is probably the best equipment for you.

	Model 1	Model 2	Model 3
Is my body secure (seat width, foot straps, belt width, padding)?	_____	_____	_____
Is it sturdy, with a rigid frame that doesn't wobble when used?	_____	_____	_____
Can I easily change the resistance while exercising?	_____	_____	_____

	Model 1	Model 2	Model 3
Is it easy to assemble (or will the dealer assemble it)?	_____	_____	_____
Is it easy to move from place to place when assembled?	_____	_____	_____
Is it easy to get on and off of?	_____	_____	_____
Does it have the gauges I want (timer, speedometer, odometer, calories used)?	_____	_____	_____
Are the gauges clear and easy to read?	_____	_____	_____
Are the gauges and controls easy to operate?	_____	_____	_____
Is the resistance knob marked so I can set it to the same place again?	_____	_____	_____
Will it fit in the space I have selected?	_____	_____	_____
Can it be adjusted to "fit" my body (seat height, frame length, footrests, stride length, handlebars)?	_____	_____	_____
Can it fit everyone who will be using it?	_____	_____	_____
Am I comfortable exercising on this equipment?	_____	_____	_____
Will I enjoy doing this activity on a regular basis?	_____	_____	_____
Does it work smoothly (no jerking or sticking)?	_____	_____	_____
Does it operate quietly?	_____	_____	_____

	Model 1	Model 2	Model 3
Are parts and service available locally?	_____	_____	_____
Does it come with a warranty? (Compare length and coverage.)	_____	_____	_____
Is shipping included in the price?	_____	_____	_____
Is it a price I can afford?	_____	_____	_____

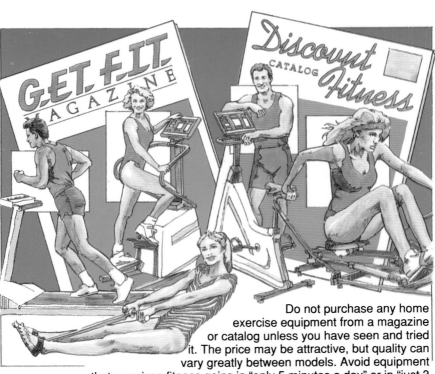

Do not purchase any home exercise equipment from a magazine or catalog unless you have seen and tried it. The price may be attractive, but quality can vary greatly between models. Avoid equipment that promises fitness gains in "only 5 minutes a day" or in "just 3 weeks." You can't get fit in such short periods.

Choosing Home Weight Training Equipment

Take this checklist to the store with you. Compare several models; put a check next to questions that you can answer "yes." The model with the most checks is probably the best equipment for you.

	Model 1	Model 2	Model 3
Is the equipment sturdy (no wobbling or loose weights)?	_____	_____	_____
Do the weights move smoothly (no sticking or jerking)?	_____	_____	_____
Are all of the exercise positions comfortable?	_____	_____	_____
Does it come with a manual?	_____	_____	_____
Is it easy to assemble?	_____	_____	_____
Is it easy to change the amount of weight (or resistance) being used?	_____	_____	_____
Is additional weight available?	_____	_____	_____
Does the equipment fit in the space I have selected?	_____	_____	_____
If it has to be attached to a wall, do I have the space available?	_____	_____	_____
If not, can I buy a special stand to attach it to?	_____	_____	_____
Does the equipment fit my body?	_____	_____	_____
Does the equipment have a padded bench?	_____	_____	_____
Can I work every major muscle group?	_____	_____	_____

	Model 1	Model 2	Model 3
Are parts and service available locally?	_____	_____	_____
Is there a warranty? (Compare length and coverage.)	_____	_____	_____
Is shipping included in the price?	_____	_____	_____
Is it a price I can afford?	_____	_____	_____

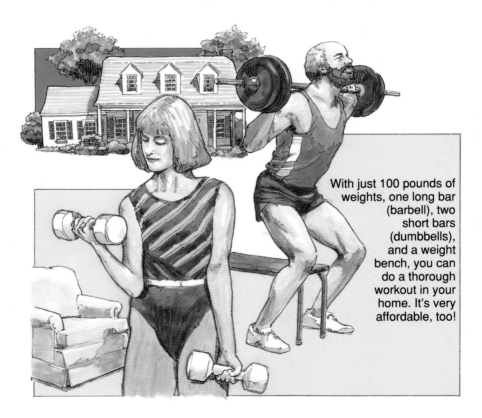

With just 100 pounds of weights, one long bar (barbell), two short bars (dumbbells), and a weight bench, you can do a thorough workout in your home. It's very affordable, too!

Choosing a
Fitness Center

Take this checklist to the fitness center with you. Compare several centers; put a check next to the questions that you can answer "yes." The center earning the most checks is probably the best one for you.

	Center 1	Center 2	Center 3
Is each member given an orientation to using the equipment?	_____	_____	_____
Is screening done on new members (health history, fitness assessment)?	_____	_____	_____
Are staff members certified in CPR?	_____	_____	_____
Are all exercise areas monitored by staff?	_____	_____	_____
Are staff involved with members in the exercise areas?	_____	_____	_____
Does the staff encourage warm-up and cool-down?	_____	_____	_____
Are members encouraged to monitor pulse rates?	_____	_____	_____
Are safety rules posted?	_____	_____	_____
Are policies, procedures, and safety guidelines in writing?	_____	_____	_____
Does the center have posted emergency procedures?	_____	_____	_____
Is the center bonded?	_____	_____	_____
Are instructors certified by ACSM (or IDEA or AFAA)?	_____	_____	_____
Is all equipment in good working order?	_____	_____	_____

	Center 1	Center 2	Center 3
Are lockers provided?	————	————	————
Do the locker rooms provide the supplies I want (soap, towels, shampoo)?	————	————	————
Is there easy access to drinking water in the exercise areas?	————	————	————
Is the center close to my home or work place?	————	————	————
Is there convenient and adequate parking?	————	————	————
If needed, is child care available?	————	————	————
Are aerobics and other classes appropriate for me?	————	————	————
Would I be comfortable exercising alongside the other members here?	————	————	————
Are staff friendly?	————	————	————
Does the center invite prospective members to a free workout?	————	————	————
Is the center manager certified by ACSM?	————	————	————
Do staff monitor progress with follow-up fitness testing?	————	————	————
Do staff encourage keeping records of workouts?	————	————	————
Is there a variety of equipment?	————	————	————
Is there enough equipment available at the time of day I'll be using it?	————	————	————

	Center 1	Center 2	Center 3
Are locker rooms and fitness areas clean, well-lit, secure, and well-ventilated?	_____	_____	_____
Is there a trial or introductory period?	_____	_____	_____
Can I afford the membership fee?	_____	_____	_____

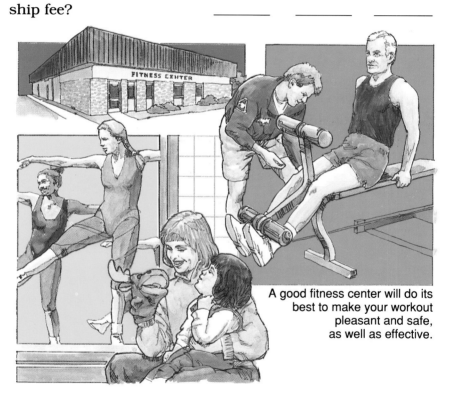

A good fitness center will do its best to make your workout pleasant and safe, as well as effective.

Choosing a Fitness Book
or Video

Evaluate books and videos according to this checklist; place a check next to each question that you can answer "yes." The book or video with the most checks is probably your best buy.

	Book or Video 1	Book or Video 2	Book or Video 3
Does the author have appropriate credentials in the fitness field (or has he or she been assisted by someone who does)?	_____	_____	_____
Is the book or video appropriate for my age, health status, and fitness level?	_____	_____	_____
Does it encourage the safe exercises in chapter 4?	_____	_____	_____
Does it encourage me to develop all components of fitness?	_____	_____	_____
Does it encourage me to warm up before exercise and cool down after?	_____	_____	_____
Does it follow the guidelines for developing cardiorespiratory fitness (see p. 94)?	_____	_____	_____
Does it encourage me to monitor my heart rate during aerobic activity?	_____	_____	_____
Does it follow the guidelines for developing muscular strength and endurance (see p. 98)?	_____	_____	_____
Does it encourage me to stop doing anything that hurts my body?	_____	_____	_____

	Book or Video 1	Book or Video 2	Book or Video 3
Is it free from claims about spot reduction, cellulite reduction, and quick weight loss?	_____	_____	_____
Is it free from claims about "no-sweat" workouts, and quick fitness?	_____	_____	_____
Is it free of any promotion of special products, devices, or nutritional supplements?	_____	_____	_____
Is this a workout I can do on a regular basis?	_____	_____	_____
Can I afford the price?	_____	_____	_____

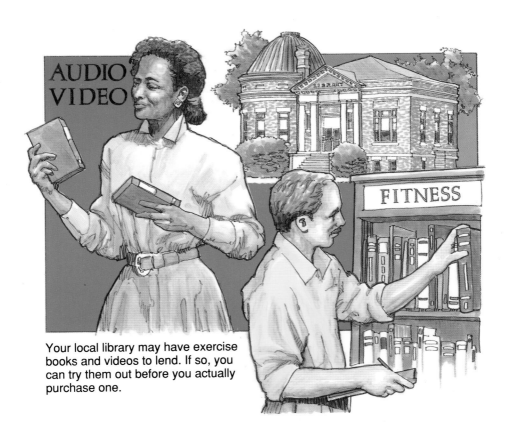

Your local library may have exercise books and videos to lend. If so, you can try them out before you actually purchase one.

Other Fitness Resources

There are many reputable nonprofit and government organizations that provide fitness and health information to the public. This information is prepared by experts and is often provided to individuals free or at low cost. Call or write to the organization.

American College of Sports Medicine
401 W. Michigan St.
Indianapolis, IN 46202-3233
(317) 637-9200

> The American College of Sports Medicine has more than 13,000 members in 50 countries around the globe working in a vast array of medical specialties, allied health professions, and scientific disciplines. Contact ACSM to receive information about publications and educational materials prepared expressly for the lay public by the leading experts in sports medicine and exercise science.

American Heart Association
7320 Greenville Ave.
Dallas, TX 75231
(213) 373-6300

> Information on heart disease, nutrition, exercise, and smoking (check your local office of the association for information first).

President's Council on Physical Fitness and Sports
450 Fifth St., NW, Suite 7103
Washington, DC 20001
(202) 272-3421

> Information on walking, jogging, and exercise and weight control. Fitness fact sheets for seniors, youth, and adults.
>
>   The President's Council also offers the Presidential Sports Award, which provides a challenge to improve fitness through regular participation in any of 49 activities.

National Association of Governors' Councils on Physical
  Fitness and Sports (NAGCPFS)
Pan American Plaza
201 S. Capitol Avenue
Suite 440
Indianapolis, IN 46225
(317) 237-5630

In addition to the President's Council just described, many states have Governor's Councils
on Physical Fitness and Sports. The purpose of
the NAGCPFS is to promote, support, and unify
those state councils. Check with the NAGCPFS
to learn whether your state has a council.

A Final Word

The ACSM Fitness Program is designed to start you on a safe,
sensible road to better fitness, and we've included information
to keep you moving even beyond the ACSM program. We hope
that your journey to a healthier you will never end. Good luck!

Index

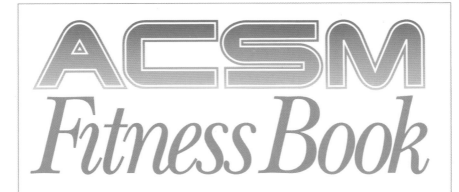

Special Quantity Discounts

Would you like to make copies of this practical and informative book available to your employees, colleagues, or clients? Human Kinetics Publishers offers a special discount schedule that makes the *ACSM Fitness Book* a unique and affordable option for you!

Discounts start with orders of 10 copies or more. Just call our order department at the telephone numbers below and ask about our special discounts for quantities of the *ACSM Fitness Book*.

Place your credit card order today! (VISA, AMEX, MC)
TOLL FREE: U.S. (800) 747-4457 • Canada (800) 465-7301
OR: U.S. (217) 351-5076 • Canada (519) 944-7774
FAX: U.S. (217) 351-2674 • Canada (519) 944-7614

Human Kinetics Publishers

AMW-1217